6 weeks to
SENSATIONAL SKIN

6 weeks to SENSATIONAL SKIN

Dr. Loretta's
BEAUTY CAMP HANDBOOK
for Your
FRESHEST FACE

LORETTA CIRALDO, MD

VOLUNTARY PROFESSOR OF DERMATOLOGY,
UNIVERSITY OF MIAMI
MILLER SCHOOL OF MEDICINE

RODALE

© 2006 by Loretta Ciraldo, MD

Book design by Anthony Serge

Library of Congress Cataloging-in-Publication Data

Ciraldo, Loretta.
    6 weeks to sensational skin : Dr. Loretta's beauty camp handbook for your freshest face / Loretta Ciraldo.
        p.   cm.
    Includes bibliographical references and index.
    ISBN-13 978–1–59486–475–9   hardcover
    ISBN-10 1–59486–475–6   hardcover
    1. Skin—Care and hygiene   2. Face—Care and hygiene.
    3. Beauty, Personal.   4. Cosmetics.   I. Title.   II. Title: Six weeks to sensational skin.
    RL87.C547   2006
    614.4'323—dc22   2006020892

Distributed to the book trade by Holtzbrinck Publishers

2   4   6   8   10   9   7   5   3   1   hardcover

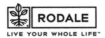

To my mother, Yolanda Bello Caruso,
who taught me that nothing is impossible.
I will try to earn my place in heaven with you.

Contents

Acknowledgments

As I gather my thoughts about who to thank for their help in making this book a reality, the list grows surprisingly long. It begins with devoted teachers, who really can change the world through the students they nurture and inspire. Having grown up in a time when it was unusual for a woman—especially one from my socioeconomic background—to become a doctor, I owe tremendous gratitude to the teachers who dared to encourage me to pursue whatever my heart desired. Without the great fortune of being able to study within the New York public school system, including the City University of New York (Hunter College) and the State University of New York (Downstate Medical School), I would not be where I am today. I applaud all those who work to give life and quality to public education.

Then there are the men who seem to have been born into this world to foster change, in dramatic and positive ways. If they are blessed with wisdom and respect for mankind, they can elevate fields like dermatology to new planes. Those who are fortunate to spend time in their company will be forever enriched by the experience. Such was the case for me many years ago, when I got to work with John Parrish, MD, and Rox Anderson, MD. And I can't forget Michael Fisher, MD, who was instrumental in helping so many of us residents to become not only outstanding dermatologists but respectful and caring physicians.

I also have learned so much from those I was meant to teach. It is a pleasure to thank all of the residents and students I have had the honor of instructing during the last couple of decades, with a special nod to Douglas Rosen, MD, Alan Halpern, MD, and Warren Heymann, MD.

Of course, professional success and recognition would mean little without personal happiness. I am blessed to have people in my life who give me joy every day. Robert, my loving husband of nearly 30 years, and Gina Yolanda, Daniel Guy, Katrina Jeanette, and Liza Rose, our wonderful and inspiring children, are my reason for being. I thank God for them every day. My brothers Michael and Joe make Mommy proud of us as she watches on. My large, extended Italian-American family is the best any woman could ever hope for.

I thank Don, who so many years ago caught me on air and recognized a talent I never knew I had; Leslee, who after just a brief meeting became instrumental in helping me pursue my goals; and Yvonne, a true friend who has shown me how resilient the human spirit can be. Giovanna and Alfio, you have helped us live the dream. My staff—Sharon, Lana, Rebecca, Chris, Maria, Dyana, Zinga, Ingrid, Maryanne, Holly, and Drusilla (and, of course, Patricia and Britt)—makes life that much easier for me. I realize being with me is never routine; I'm grateful for your flexibility.

Neeti Madan, my book agent, has an amazing balance of

grace and intellect. She made this project seem achievable right from the beginning. Susan Berg, my editor, is a patient, supportive, and talented human being; I thank her for everything. My thanks, too, to the supporting cast at Rodale—Lois Hazel, Rachelle Vander Schaaf, Susan Eugster, Tara Long, Trish Field, and Anthony Serge—each of whom did their part to create a book that I'm proud of.

And thank you, dear reader, for without your interest this book would not exist.

Orientation

A Welcome Letter from Dr. Loretta

Hello, campers. Welcome to Beauty Camp! It's the culmination of 25 years of examining and treating thousands of women (and men) who have come to me with high hopes of developing a plan for having better skin. I love what I do; dermatology is my job and my passion. Give me a skin-care problem, and I want to solve it. Ask me what I think of your overall appearance and the quality of your skin, and I can't help but be honest.

Like so many doctors, though, I've found that the traditional practice of medicine can be a frustrating enterprise. I am bound by terrible time constraints. You make an appointment to see me. You wait—sometimes weeks—for the appointment day to come. Once inside my office, you wait some more. After all that waiting—and more waiting—an office visit may last all of 10 minutes.

As a responsible physician, I'm obligated to address your most pressing needs—things that may truly be problematic or life threatening—first. But what about everything else? Even though I squeeze as much into each office visit as I can and have printed lots of handouts and brochures for my patients to take with them, I often wish I could help more.

What would be my dream? It's a little revolutionary, but I've always imagined a more relaxed setting in which I could relate to my patients as friends. We could spend more time together, perhaps the equivalent of a dozen regular office visits. In that informal atmosphere, I wouldn't just look at your skin, mole by mole. I'd see a bigger picture. I would share the knowledge and advice that I've accumulated over the years—but I wouldn't do all the talking, either. You and I would have a more satisfying, in-depth exchange. We'd laugh; we'd make some confessions; we'd brainstorm. It would be fun—and more rewarding than an in-and-out appointment.

And I'd do my best to answer all of your questions. What could you improve, and what should you leave alone? How far can you go—and how do you know when you're there? These are the sorts of personal decisions all of us make, consciously or unconsciously. We want to look better, but not weirdly altered. We want to appear healthy and youthful, but we don't want our features stretched and peeled into oblivion. Gosh, we just want to look like ourselves—only better.

Ideally, we would have a series of six weekly meetings. At our first meeting, we'd talk about your face and what you might want to improve. I'd tell you a bit about the structure and com- position of skin. We'd spend the next 2 weeks evaluating your current skin-care regimen to determine what's working for you and what isn't, as well as whether any particular products may be irritating your skin or clogging your pores. Over the subse- quent 4 weeks, we would test new products and ingredients, constructing a skin-care routine that would leave your skin looking sensational—with fewer fine lines, smaller pores, and less redness, blotchiness, and discoloration.

If you like the sound of this, then I hope you'll keep reading! Because what I've just described to you is the philosophy behind Beauty Camp. I'd love to help!

I've written this book as a way to offer a fun, reinvigorating approach to good skin care—and to share my many experiences and insights along the way. Over the years, I've worked with people of all ages, ethnicities, and skin types—patients, family members, friends, and neighbors. To this day, whenever I meet a new person and see a new face, I can't help but mentally perform a makeover. Part of me is still the young girl who cut the hair of everyone in the family, who studied all the beauty magazines, who loved nothing more than experimenting with skin-care products or applying a girlfriend's makeup.

When I decided to study premed, my Italian-American mother was a little mystified. Why would I bother with being a doctor? As far as my mom could tell, I already had a calling as a beautician. The years have passed, and I continue to love helping people look better, feel better, and enjoy their appearance—and themselves. My friends and my children can tell you that.

This book combines my playful and serious sides. Everything that I'll share with you has a solid medical and scientific foundation. I should mention, too, that most of the products and ingredients I'll recommend in this book have been tested on my own skin first. I'm blessed (or cursed) with incredibly sensitive skin and a propensity for scarring and discoloration. So I can assure you, as my own best guinea pig, that if something has proven safe and effective on me, it could be a jewel for you and others.

You could breeze through this book in a night or a week—or linger over the exercises for 2 or 3 months. To me, 6 weeks is the perfect amount of time to educate yourself, experiment, evaluate, and get feedback from family and friends. It's also the perfect amount of time for me to teach you how to look at your face and skin as I would. You'll discover new things about yourself and learn to care for your skin in the best possible way. I must warn you, though: Some of your most basic notions about skin care are about to be overturned!

YOUR SKIN-CARE PERSONALITY

Over the years, I've noticed that the people who come to my practice for skin-care advice and procedures tend to fall into several categories, each of which reflects a general personality type. For instance, a diehard skin-care junkie will try almost anything—and spend almost anything—to look her best. She's an optimist, really. She is convinced that her appearance is under her control and always improvable. The problem is, she's prone to going overboard and doing too much.

The pessimist has a different problem. She's convinced that most products and procedures are a hoax and that improving the appearance of her skin is hopeless. She may miss out on the chance to look better, even when she easily could.

Most of us fall into a third category: We're willing to try new things, but we aren't sure how far to go or how much to spend. We're a little skeptical, too: Do those miracle creams and lotions really work?

Many of us have dropped hundreds if not thousands of dollars on cosmetics that promise to clear, cleanse, tone, smooth, and otherwise improve our skin. It's true that these days, we can dramatically alter its appearance without scalpels and plastic surgery or even needles and Botox. But that means choosing from a dizzying array of products. Which ones really work? And do they work for everyone? Can skin care be one-size-fits-all?

And what about all those products at department-store cosmetics counters—the ones that cost a small fortune? Are they that much better than less expensive drugstore brands?

Perhaps you're almost a cynic; your instincts tell you that most product claims are a scam. In your view, women are the targets of huge marketing campaigns that attempt to make us feel unattractive and insecure while they promise to transform us—if only we'll buy whatever it is that they're offering.

At Beauty Camp, you'll learn how to read the labels of products before you buy them. You'll seek out beneficial ingredients to put on your face instead of buying into a promise—or a texture or smell. You'll discover that, although many manufacturers want you to buy into their critical, almost sacred skin-care systems, the order in which you apply creams and lotions to your face doesn't matter. (The smallest molecules are absorbed first, regardless of the order in which products are applied.) You'll finally free yourself from the tyranny of skin typing: Well-formulated skin-care products are generally safe for everyone, whether your skin is dry (meaning that it lacks good hydration) or oily (it makes too much sebum)—or both.

We'll also spend some time talking about the new procedures that are available in a cosmetic dermatologist's office. If there's something you've seriously considered, you need to know how to go about finding a good doctor and then getting an effective treatment. And how much should you pay? You may be worried about your budget—and with good reason. Some procedures can be a serious drain on the pocketbook.

Then again, maybe you don't see yourself as the cosmetic procedure sort. Your friends are trying lasers and glycolic peels and other expensive in-office treatments, but you've resisted them so far. You might perceive yourself as more "natural" than that, or simply less vain.

To be honest, I'd encourage everyone to try at-home treatments first. Many of these produce results immediately—and some offer more profound improvements when used regularly for 6 weeks.

THE UNINVITED ELEMENTS:
TO CHANGE OR NOT TO CHANGE?

This brings us back to a question I asked a bit earlier: What could you improve, and what should you leave alone? The truth is, even if you've inherited the greatest skin in the world and taken good care of it, there are bound to be things about your face that trouble you.

Before we explore these questions further, let me tell you something. It's more of a confession, really: Some people think I talk too fast. Well, it's true. Words just spill out of my mouth sometimes, and I've been known to interrupt people on occasion. I've even done this on TV. (Once I talked right over Barbara Walters—like a steamroller.) I'm mindful of this tendency of mine, and I do try to be as polite as possible. But talking fast is part of who I am. It reflects my personality and my New York origin.

It's funny. For 20-plus years, I've lived in Miami. I've raised four children there. I run a busy private practice there. I'm a voluntary professor of dermatology at the University of Miami; in 2005, I was elected president of the Dade County Medical Association. I've also developed a private-label skin-care line. Of course, I'm very proud of all these accomplishments. But no matter how far I go, the New York accent and fast-talking style stay with me.

I suppose I could do something about it. I could train myself to change pace—to erase my past from my present. But guess what? I can't imagine being any different. Erase my Queens accent from my voice, and you'd erase part of me.

This gets to the heart of my philosophy about appearance. I don't have a perfect face. I don't have perfect skin, either. As I said before, I have extremely sensitive skin; if I just think about something stressful, red blotches appear all over my face. I've been swollen and even bruised after trying a new scrub, and I've broken out in bad acne from using certain shampoos. And even though I'm a dermatologist, I have sun damage like almost everyone else.

As for bone structure and symmetry, my facial features are not in balance. My forehead is narrow; my mouth, wide; my eyes, too small (I'm sure they are). And now, at age 53, I've noticed that my eyebrows seem to be trying to move down to meet the bottom of my face, and my chin is puckering up on me.

But it's my face. It's the face that I have been carrying

around with me every day for all these years. It's the face that grew up and went to college and medical school in New York City. It's the face that my husband, Rob, fell in love with. It's the face that my four children know and count on. It's my face and nobody else's.

I've never had a face-lift, though I do use Botox—just a few injections right below my hairline to raise my otherwise fallen brow. It's one of my Uninvited Elements, or what I call UEs for short. If your cheeks sag a little at the jawline, then those sags are UEs. Droopy eyelids and laugh lines are UEs; so are thinning lips, double chins, and liver spots.

Some UEs add character and beauty to your face, while others detract. In Week #1 of Beauty Camp, I'll ask you to do an honest assessment of your own UEs and help you decide which you'd like to change and which you don't mind keeping just as they are. To me, my eyebrows are like my Queens accent: Would I still be Loretta if the sags went away completely?

AGE IS WHAT YOU MAKE IT

Getting to know your UEs—and your skin in general—is one thing. Getting to know your expectations is another. But it's just as essential. What I expect to look like, especially as I grow older, may not be the same as what you expect. So while we're discussing the particulars of spots and pores and fine lines, it might be smart to give some consideration to the bigger picture.

In my cosmetic dermatology practice, a great majority of the patients who come to see me are seeking advice about how to reduce or reverse the changes that occur with time and age.

Time passes, and aging is inevitable. Yet in our culture, we tend to approach it with a sense of disappointment, sometimes even dread. How did it happen? What went awry? We may feel young on the inside, so why don't we look that way on the outside?

I have many thoughts about this—and much to say. To begin with: What is "old age" supposed to look like? What should we see in the mirror at age 60, 70, or 80? Can we live with those changes?

To me, that's one of the wonderful things about getting older: The angst fades as you become accustomed to yourself— a bit more comfortable and relaxed in your own skin or, perhaps, simply resigned to it. This is particularly true if you've achieved some of your goals in life and reached a level of happiness and satisfaction. When you're proud of what you've accomplished, it's easier to stop wishing you looked like this person or that.

My own face is pretty youthful, though seasoned. (My kids would say that it's vintage.) At some point in life, it became like an old friend. I am loyal to that old friend—and I take care of it.

The fashion designer Coco Chanel once said that we get the face we deserve at 50. Is this true? After all, a number of factors determine how we age. While some—like nutrition, fitness, and environment—are within our control, others—like genetics, hormones, and, of course, gravity—are not. There are women born with great skin and a tendency not to get craggy; women with an underlying bone structure that prevents sunken, crinkled cheeks; women with a natural hormone balance that keeps their skin looking smooth and youthful. I also know women who have eaten well, exercised, and protected their skin from the sun; now, in middle age, they are reaping the benefits.

What about those of us who have not been blessed with good genes or who have been less than attentive to our skin? No matter what your age, you can take steps to restore and protect your skin's appearance and resilience. They're not drastic measures, either. Simply revamping your skin-care regimen can make a huge difference. Many of my patients tell me that their skin doesn't look as healthy as it once did, even though they're using the same products that they have for years. Often that's precisely the problem!

As your skin changes with time and age, your skin-care regimen needs to change, as well. That's why, during the second week of Beauty Camp, we'll be collecting all the products that you use on your face and hair and going through them one by one to decide what you should keep and what you should part with. From there, we'll discuss and sample new (and not so new) products, building a skin-care regimen that's just right for you. It may not stop the clock, but it certainly will slow it down a bit.

Little Things Mean a Lot

It may seem clichéd, but I genuinely believe that so much of appearance is making the most of what you've got—of putting your best face forward. Have you ever gathered a small bunch of flowers or ironed the cloth napkins to make dinner just a little more special? That's how I feel about appearance. I'm more comfortable and relaxed if I've put forth a little effort.

When I say a "little," I'm thinking smart and simple changes. It isn't about undergoing dramatic alterations to look

20 years younger. After all, you wouldn't rush out to buy new wine glasses when friends are dropping by; the ones you have on hand will do just fine. In fact, I still am pretty sentimental about a set of glasses we bought on a family vacation about a decade ago. The gold trim is wearing off, but if I put other gold-toned pieces on the table, the glasses look almost regal.

The same principle applies to personal appearance. A smile can brighten a face like a bouquet of flowers does a table. In fact, quite a few studies have proven this: Smiling women are perceived as vastly more attractive than non-smiling women, regardless of other facial features, body type, and even age. In one study presented in the *Journal of Personality and Social Psychology*, older women shown smiling were perceived as more attractive than younger women who were not. A smile turns out to be the real face-lift!

And if that's all it takes to look your best—healthy, rested, and youthful—isn't it worth a try? That's one of the most important lessons of Beauty Camp: Whether it's buying a new pillowcase or learning a new technique for applying eyeliner, often the smallest changes produce the biggest results.

Time to Get Started!

When you opened this book, you arrived at Beauty Camp. Come alone or with your daughter or sister or a few friends— the ones who can be helpful without being cruel, the ones who are also interested in looking good and taking care of their skin. Organize an afternoon or an evening when you can meet together. Or plan to take some time for yourself. I'll stick with you—don't worry.

Together, we'll cry with laughter and commiserate. We'll trade secrets and share makeup. We'll memorize the Beauty Camp code of conduct. We'll tell scary stories by the campfire. Just like during those halcyon days of summers long ago, when you were a girl at summer camp, you'll enjoy moments of self-discovery. You'll effortlessly absorb practical information and relax into a skin-care routine that's designed just for you. At the end of 6 weeks, you'll leave Beauty Camp looking and feeling better—with more confidence and a stronger sense of who you are.

This book contains hundreds of tips—the equivalent of dozens of office visits. As your beauty camp counselor, I intend to give you exactly the same advice that I give my own daughters and friends, as well as my patients. I'll be frank with you and generous with ideas, but also practical and budget conscious. I believe in commonsense approaches and trying at-home treatments before jumping into in-office procedures that are expensive and sometimes risky.

Come to Beauty Camp, and you'll figure out what you can fix and what you can't—and what you shouldn't. You'll learn some very simple (and proven) skin-care strategies that you may not be aware of. For example, did you know that sleeping on your face can cause grooves, lines, and puffy eyes? That washing your face with tepid water—never hot—can reduce redness and prevent broken capillaries? That changing your shampoo or conditioner might put an end to acne?

These and other Camp Rules will guide you through the basics of good skin care, which will help you look better and healthier at any age. At the end of each week of Beauty Camp, we'll review these rules and why they matter. Along the way, there will be lessons to learn, activities to do, and new habits to form. For some, this won't require much effort. For others, it could be more difficult. Old habits really do die hard! That's why I believe it's so important for you to understand not just what you should change, but why.

After 6 weeks at Beauty Camp, you should see a noticeable improvement in your skin. Fine lines and pores will be less visible; any redness, blotchiness, or discoloration should fade. If you're looking for even more dramatic results—or if you're just curious—you may want to read the special section at the end of the book, where I give the lowdown on an array of popular (and often effective) in-office procedures—from glycolic peels and lasers to Botox and Restylane.

It's never too late to try something new—to reinvent yourself, even a little bit. It's never too late to take another look at yourself in the mirror and see what you might want to change. Your skin is constantly changing anyway; why not make the most of it?

—*Dr. Loretta*

CHECKLIST:

WHAT TO BRING TO BEAUTY CAMP

Before you head to Beauty Camp, you'll want to gather a few essential items. The following list may seem odd to you; just like Beauty Camp, it's full of surprises. And there's barely a skin-care product on it!

☐ **Digital camera or Polaroid camera with film.** So many of us make the mistake of using magnifying mirrors, assuming they reveal how we really look in the world. The problem is, nobody ever stands that close to you with a magnifier—except maybe your dermatologist! A candid (or semicandid) photograph will give you a more objective and accurate perspective on how you look to others. It also will provide a record of how you look at the beginning of Beauty Camp that you can compare to another one after 6 weeks.

☐ **Soft, 400-thread-count, all-cotton pillowcase.** Think how much time you spend with your face on a pillow. That's why it's essential to find yourself a surface that's much kinder to cuddle up with for 8 straight hours. And the softer, the better! It will cause much less irritation to your skin, particularly if you are using Retin-A or any strong creams at bedtime.

☐ **New or (freshly cleaned) washcloth.** Bacteria will grow on anything, but a damp washcloth or sponge really is a perfect environment for cultures to thrive in. So if you like to wash your face with a cloth or sponge, be sure it's new or clean before you use it. Otherwise, you could be causing problems for your skin.

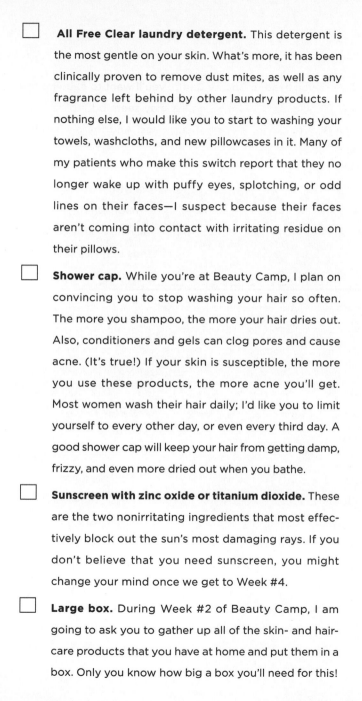

☐ **All Free Clear laundry detergent.** This detergent is the most gentle on your skin. What's more, it has been clinically proven to remove dust mites, as well as any fragrance left behind by other laundry products. If nothing else, I would like you to start to washing your towels, washcloths, and new pillowcases in it. Many of my patients who make this switch report that they no longer wake up with puffy eyes, splotching, or odd lines on their faces—I suspect because their faces aren't coming into contact with irritating residue on their pillows.

☐ **Shower cap.** While you're at Beauty Camp, I plan on convincing you to stop washing your hair so often. The more you shampoo, the more your hair dries out. Also, conditioners and gels can clog pores and cause acne. (It's true!) If your skin is susceptible, the more you use these products, the more acne you'll get. Most women wash their hair daily; I'd like you to limit yourself to every other day, or even every third day. A good shower cap will keep your hair from getting damp, frizzy, and even more dried out when you bathe.

☐ **Sunscreen with zinc oxide or titanium dioxide.** These are the two nonirritating ingredients that most effectively block out the sun's most damaging rays. If you don't believe that you need sunscreen, you might change your mind once we get to Week #4.

☐ **Large box.** During Week #2 of Beauty Camp, I am going to ask you to gather up all of the skin- and hair-care products that you have at home and put them in a box. Only you know how big a box you'll need for this!

Week #1

Arriving at Camp

This week's agenda:
Learning to see your face the way I do

Your face travels around with you, like a billboard for your spirit. It vividly expresses your attitudes about yourself and the world around you. In years of treating patients in my cosmetic dermatology practice, I can't help but notice that people tend to consider matters of the face and appearance the same way they approach other aspects of life: Optimists think they look a whole lot better than they really do; pessimists find problems everywhere.

At any age, we rarely see ourselves objectively. It becomes even more difficult as we grow older. We might toy with the idea of getting a face-lift, but we haven't changed our hairdos in decades. We might brood about our wrinkles, but we remain competely attached to—almost sentimental about—the skin-care products and regimens that we've been using for years.

Some people obsess over one particular flaw that they believe overshadows all others and demands attention. Patients come to my office with odd complaints quite often. For example, they see lines that are barely noticeable in normal daylight or to the naked eye. In their minds, minor imperfections like these seem monstrous and unacceptable.

When a patient focuses on an almost invisible detail—a few thin lines above her lips, pores that seem too large, a chicken pox scar from childhood—then I know she's been examining herself with a high-powered magnifying mirror. She isn't seeing her whole face anymore. She's looking at herself one feature at a time, and her pores look like craters on the moon.

In reality, this patient is expressing a desire to look better. She bought that magnifying mirror for a reason: She wants to improve her appearance. But the mirror isn't guiding her to the details she needs to notice. It has blurred the big picture—and any sense of objectivity along with it.

Professionally, it's not appropriate for me to mention something about a patient's appearance that doesn't seem to be bothering her. It's my job to address her concerns, not mine. She might have a large *solar lentigo*, or age spot, on her left cheek (probably caused by ultraviolet rays penetrating her car's window while she's driving). But since this is a cosmetic issue and not a health-related one, I won't ask my patient if she'd consider treating the age spot with hydroquinone or a series of glycolic acid peels.

As we talk a bit more, I might notice that her teeth have gotten yellow and wonder why she hasn't tried a tooth whitener. (For many people, even commercial products, like Crest Whitestrips, are really effective.) I also might wonder why she chose that shade of lipstick, because it seems all wrong for her complexion. I might contemplate her hairstyle and imagine other styles that would frame her face better. (Women tend to think that short hair is more becoming to older faces, but often it isn't.)

This is how I see my patients' faces—and how I want you to see your own. It's time to put away the magnifying mirror and get out the camera. We're going to take your Orientation photos.

CAMP ACTIVITY #1
TAKING YOUR ORIENTATION PHOTOS

Right now you might be thinking, *Photos? She didn't say we'd need to take photos!* Most of us dislike going in front of a camera. Somehow, the image we see in the picture never quite resembles or reflects the person we believe ourselves to be. Also, we grow so accustomed to staring at ourselves in the bathroom mirror—straight on, in a certain light, in a certain pose—that viewing ourselves at new angles can be almost jarring: *Is that really me? It can't be!*

But if we don't learn to look at our faces bravely, we're in danger of elephant-in-the-room syndrome. All of us have known women who aren't addressing the central issue of their appearance—whether it's blotchy skin or a big age spot. They just don't notice what seems so apparent to everyone else. Is such self-scrutiny too painful? Too complicated? Too narcissistic?

It shouldn't be any of these things. Rather, it should be about honesty—about learning to really see ourselves. Photographs objectively show the parts of our faces that we try very hard to conceal or ignore. The more objective we can be about our appearance, the better able we are to improve it or embrace it—to simply say, "That's who I am. And I can live with it."

To get an adequate record of your face, you will need at least three snapshots. Your spouse or child could take them, or your mother or sister. It's a good idea to find somebody with whom you are comfortable, who doesn't make you feel overly self-conscious. You could take the photos yourself by setting your camera's timer or photographing your reflection in a mirror. (If choosing the latter, just be sure not to use the flash.)

If you are among a group of women who've decided to attend Beauty Camp together, you could take pictures of each other at your first meeting or invite a photographer to join your group for the night. But the setting should be relaxed and comfortable.

Polaroids are easy and instantly gratifying, though if you have a digital camera and a color printer, they can work just as well. Be sure to stand in decent light indoors or in the shade on a sunny day outdoors. The light should be bright enough to reveal your lines and grooves, but not so bright that it washes them out and hides them. Try various natural poses—talking, smiling, laughing, listening. Turn your face away from the camera for a few shots. A profile shot would be good, along with a three-quarter.

The point is not to capture your face at the best angle or advantage or to look in your photos exactly as you do in the bathroom mirror. (You already know how you look in the bathroom mirror!) The point is to provide an accurate record of what you truly look like as you go about your day-to-day routine. In many cases, these would be the kind of pictures that you'd rip up when they come back from the photo shop (or the ones you'd delete from the memory card of your digital camera).

From your shoot, choose at least three photos—a view of your left side, one of your right side, and a straight frontal portrait. These snapshots will be invaluable to you. Like a videotape of your golf swing or an underwater film of your swimming strokes, these images are meant to help you see yourself clearly, as you look to others. As we progress through the rest of Beauty Camp, they'll serve as a record of your appearance at the beginning.

You don't need to show them to anyone, either. They are intended for your eyes only. At the end of the book, I've set aside a few blank pages where you can glue or tape your photos if you wish. That way, as we continue through Beauty Camp, you can flip back to your photos and study and reflect upon your progress.

CAMP ACTIVITY #2
ANALYZING YOUR ORIENTATION PHOTOS

In order to look at your face objectively—rather than through the lens of the relationship that you've had with yourself and your appearance over the years—you might need a bit of practice. Actors know how to do this, as do models. But don't worry. I'm not trying to turn you into a supermodel or pushing you to a surgeon's office. I just want to show you how to look at yourself and recognize your best features, as well as any Uninvited Elements. (For a refresher on the UEs, see page 6 of the Orientation.)

I have two techniques that might help you overcome any psychological and emotional impediments to objectivity. One is to imagine that you're looking at a stranger's face rather than your own. The other is to imagine that it is not a photograph at all but a painting—a portrait by Picasso. Then you can see the shapes, lines, contours, and asymmetry of your face without judging it as beautiful or youthful. We aren't critiquing the image at this point. It's a painting, a work of art.

Study the eyes and nose. Look at the shape of the chin, the structure of the brows. From a frontal view, notice whether the face is symmetrical from side to side. In other words, are the right and left halves of the face almost mirror images?

Most faces are a little off-kilter. As a matter of fact, if you look at my photo on the front cover, you'll see that my right eye is significantly smaller than my left. With the creative use of makeup, I'm able to make them appear about equal in size. As a rule of thumb, symmetry is considered more attractive than asymmetry. But I certainly don't consider myself unattractive!

Now let's look for vertical symmetry, or balance. A sense of proportion is another commonly accepted aspect of what is generally defined as "beauty." It is how cosmetic surgeons are trained to look at faces—they even measure features with a ruler to assess proportion and balance. Is the forehead as long as the chin, or is one shorter than the other? Is the upper lip long enough? Does the nose seem to be in pleasing balance with the rest of the face, or does one feature seem too small or too large? (It is possible to have too small a nose!)

Which are the best features? What could be done to enhance them? Here's the idea: If you like your eyes best, then you might want to put more effort into minimizing any crow's-feet. If your nose is your favorite, you might want to pay closer attention to the skin there. Are there any clogged pores or red bumps you could easily fix?

What's Your Line?

Let's talk about the general quality of your skin. Do you see any redness or dark spots that make the color and tone seem uneven or mottled? And what about the pores—are they clean and clear? (This might be difficult to assess in a photograph, although clogged pores can cause bumps on the surface of the skin that detract from its appearance.) Also notice the surface of the skin. Is it dull and flaky or glowing and fresh?

Like most women, you probably have been led to believe that you must determine whether your skin is "dry" or "oily." The truth is, skin that is palpably oily, with excess sebum (oil from the pores), can also become red and scaly—especially in the creases around your nose.

Lines are the next thing to look for. Our faces become less smooth and more shadowy as we get older. For the most part, it's the result of structural changes in the skin over time. All the crags and sags and crow's-feet have specific medical names. For our purposes, all you need to remember is that dermatologists categorize facial lines as either *dynamic* or *static*.

Dynamic lines result from facial expressions and habitual movements, like frowning or smoking cigarettes. Static lines are the product of time, gravity, and the loss of collagen and other structural supports in the skin layers. These are lines that remain on the face even when it's at rest.

A furrowed brow and crow's-feet are dynamic, while a sagging jawline is static. Those deep lines that run from the nose to the sides of the mouth—called *nasolabial folds*—can be either static or dynamic. Sometimes a set of grooves droops from the corners of the mouth. They're known as *marionette lines*, and they also can be static or dynamic.

How about small vertical lines running upward from the upper lip? Their technical name—which doesn't sound all that technical at all—is *smoker's lines*. Since some women get them whether or not they smoke, in this book I simply will call them *lip lines*.

In almost any light, deep grooves can cast shadows that may run across the forehead, between the brows, or along the sides of the cheeks. They may form what looks like a perpetual "frown" around the mouth.

What about shadows around the eyes? Some are caused by droopy lids; others, by thinning skin. Capillaries beneath the skin can break and leak tiny amounts of blood, leading to the appearance of dark circles.

Before you get depressed about all this, I want to share some encouraging news: It's possible to minimize, if not eliminate, undereye circles with certain at-home skin-care formulations. Both dynamic and static lines can improve quite dramatically, too, with the right regimen of brand-name products—no surgery necessary. As for redness, age spots, and other stains, even they will fade and perhaps completely disappear with proper care and a little diligence on your part.

Ask for a Second Opinion

If you are willing to share your pictures with a fellow Beauty Camper, family member, or friend, find someone you trust—

maybe someone who has a good eye for detail. Keep in mind that you aren't asking this person to critique your appearance as you sit across from her (or him) and gaze directly into her eyes. Rather, the two of you will examine your photos, and you'll ask questions: "Are those bags under my eyes always there? Gosh, I never noticed those freckles before. Are they really freckles or something else, like an age spot? Does my chin really sag like that? What about my hair—does it always look straggly from the back?"

Now ask this person what she considers your UEs and which ones she thinks require improvement. Try not to take her comments personally. It may help to remember that you didn't create your face; for the most part, it was bequeathed to you.

It's amazing how differently you and this other person might view the same face. What seems like a nagging issue to you might be an asset to her. What had previously gone unnoticed by you—a few scattered blackheads, for example—might seem obvious to another. There's just nothing like getting a second opinion!

If you were coming to see me as either a patient or a friend, here's what I would look for.

- Is your face well proportioned from top to bottom?
- Does your skin have a slight glow, or is it dull?
- Is the skin tone even?
- Are there any age spots or broken blood vessels?
- Are there any signs of redness, flaking, or scales?
- Are the pores clean and clear?
- Are there dark circles under and alongside the eyes?
- Are your most prominent grooves and lines dynamic or static?

Identify Your Uninvited Elements

Using the information from your self-evaluation as well as from your second opinion (if you got one), write down your UEs in the space below. Then circle or highlight the ones you'd like to improve. This list will come in handy during the rest of Beauty Camp, as we choose the best products and treatments for your skin-care concerns.

_____   _____

_____   _____

_____   _____

_____   _____

_____   _____

_____

- -

SCARY CAMP STORY:
SLEEP DEPRIVATION

Some hairs on the back of my neck still rise when I see pictures of me at my brother Joe's wedding in the late '70s, when I was 25 years old. The wedding was in Dallas, during my internship rotation at a New York City hospital's emergency room. In order to attend the wedding, I had rearranged my schedule so that I was on call for 36 hours straight before leaving for Texas. I got on a plane at 7:00 that morning and just made the wedding ceremony, which started at noon Dallas time.

Forget the creams, the makeup, or whatever my hair was doing that day. Those things were superfluous. Without the most basic beauty tool—a good night's sleep—all else went out the window. I had almost black circles under what looked like half-shut eyes. You cannot imagine how utterly awful I looked!

Even the best skin-care regimen in the world can't compensate for not getting the proper amount of rest each night. The good news is, the opposite is just as true. Have you ever noticed how much better you look in your vacation photos, after even a few days of rest and relaxation? This is why the first rule of Beauty Camp is to increase your sleep time.

CAMP ACTIVITY #3
GETTING 30 MINUTES MORE SLEEP

If dark circles or puffy eyes made your list of UEs, I have a simple remedy that could bring about dramatic improvement. As a bonus, it will improve the general quality and appearance of your skin. I'm talking about logging more sleep time.

When you're well rested, it shows in your face. I know women who've endured extensive plastic surgery—at great pain and expense—to achieve this look. There's a much easier way, of course. You can start by modifying your sleep schedule.

What's the bare-minimum amount of sleep you should be getting? Seven hours a night. You may be getting by on less, but it isn't healthy—and it certainly isn't good for your appearance.

I have a few techniques for increasing sleep time that have worked for me and many of my pleasantly surprised patients. To start, even if you're a very busy person, try to go to bed at least 15 minutes earlier each night and wake up 15 minutes later each morning. It might seem almost impossible to lose 15 minutes of prep time in the morning, but there are a few things you can do to streamline your A.M. routine. For example, you might choose your outfit for the next day before going to bed, or shower at night instead of in the morning.

If you absolutely can't get up 15 minutes later, go to bed a half hour earlier. When I recommend this to patients, they usually tell me that this will be *really* impossible—that they'll be lucky to fall asleep at all. But with a little effort and a few changes in certain habits, they do. You can, too.

You might practice a few calming yoga poses before going to bed or read a very dull book (not this one, of course!). If you regularly consume caffeinated foods or beverages later in the day, try to cut back. I suggest not drinking coffee, tea, or cola any later than lunchtime or eating anything chocolatey in the evening. Spicy food can be stimulating, too. Wine causes some people to nod off early, while keeping others awake. (Most hard liquor has the same effect.)

Also, pay attention to your body rhythms and lifestyle patterns and how they affect your sleep habits. For example, what time of day do you exercise? Does it tend to relax you or energize you? You may need to move your workouts from evening to morning if they're keeping you awake. In my own life, I've found that even a fun, informative late-night call to one of my kids can leave me too wired to sleep.

If you can manage to squeeze another 30 minutes of sleep into your schedule—and I really urge you to try—you may be surprised by how much better you look after just several days. (You could take before-and-after pictures of this improvement alone.) A bonus: You'll feel better, too.

While we're on the subject of sleep, you may remember that your packing list for Beauty Camp included a 400-thread-count, all-cotton pillowcase. If you haven't bought one yet, I hope you'll do so now. They're sold in pairs, which is great, since you should change your pillowcase at least once a week.

Why am I making a big deal about your pillowcase? Though some women sleep on their backs, most of us lie on our stomachs or sides, with our faces scrunched against our pillows. (That's the only way I *can* sleep.) Basically, your pillowcase is like an 8-hour mask that you leave on your skin all night. So, just as you're prudent about the products you apply to your skin, you should pay attention to the surface on which you rest your face.

The cotton of your pillowcase should be fine enough and soft enough to not cause any irritation. As I mentioned in Orientation, and as we'll discuss in the weeks ahead, many of the skin-care ingredients that are most effective can cause your skin to become slightly irritated and sensitive.

When you wash your pillowcases, be sure to use All Free Clear laundry detergent—another item on your packing list. Of the detergents I've tried, this seems to be the least allergenic. Many women have told me that their sinuses and entire respiratory systems improved once they made this switch.

During Orientation, I recommended washing your pillowcases, washcloths, and towels in All Free Clear. You may want to use it for all of your washables, including your clothes.

CAMP ACTIVITY #4
TWO TRULY EFFECTIVE FACIAL EXERCISES

Before we delve into changing skin-care products or contemplate a series of at-home peels, I want you to start doing a couple of simple facial exercises. Hollywood actors and European women have talked about these exercises for years. I must admit, I was skeptical about them until I tried them. They really can work!

What convinced me to try them? A couple of years ago, I decided to add strength training to my fitness routine. But I knew from my dermatology practice that even petite women can develop significant frown lines from grimacing while they're lifting weights. When these women come into my office for Botox injections to lessen the lines, it sometimes requires two or even three times more Botox to immobilize their frown muscles, compared with the treatments for women who don't strength train. I wanted the benefits of strength training without those downsides! And I wondered: If facial movements can strengthen certain muscles, why not target the right muscles instead of the wrong ones?

So, believe it or not, I trained myself to smile instead of grimace while lifting weights. And sure enough, within a couple of months I saw improvement in my jawline. (Look at yourself in the mirror as you smile, and you'll see how your jawline really firms up.)

Not all women need facial exercises, of course. But if in examining your photographs you notice sagging around your chin and neck (for some of us, these two features become one.) or detect lines radiating from your lips, the following exercises are perfect for you. I recommend doing them daily. By the end of Beauty Camp, you will see a difference—I promise!

The smiling exercise: This is terrific for firming your jawline, minimizing lip lines, and lifting the corners of your mouth (which in itself can dramatically improve your appearance). Begin by pressing your lips tightly together to form a wide but closemouthed smile. Then slowly part your lips into a broad grin. Open your mouth wider—and wider still. Hold for 5 minutes.

I call this the smiling exercise because it engages the muscles we use when we smile. They happen to be the opposing muscles to those we use when we purse our lips—when smoking or whistling, for example. It makes physiological sense: If you strengthen one muscle group, it will diminish the lines created by the opposing muscle group. This exercise also strengthens the muscles that control the contours at the corners of your mouth. When this occurs, the corners can literally change direction—and go from a static frowning position to an uplifted one.

I suggest practicing this exercise twice a day—once in the morning and again at night. You could do it during your commute or while watching TV. If you watch yourself in a mirror, you might remind yourself of a politician faking a big smile. But you might also feel happier; smiling sure beats frowning!

The meat-chewing exercise: Extend your neck upward to tilt your head back as far as it goes comfortably. The muscle that you feel stretching is the *platysma*. Basically, your neck is made up of a series of wide bands of this muscle, running at angles between your jaw and collarbone—almost like pulleys. Keeping your head tilted back, open and close your mouth until you feel a pull on your neck. It might help to imagine that you are chewing on a piece of steak.

Do this exercise for a minimum of 5 minutes in the morning and 5 minutes at night, or whenever your schedule allows you to squeeze in a full 10 minutes. I know that 10 minutes of chewing a piece of nonexistent steak may seem tedious, but the payoff is well worth the effort. You'll strengthen and firm your chin and jawline and smooth your neck.

My former hairdresser, Stanley, who worked on everyone's hair in the heyday of Miami Beach, had a favorite client named Ginger Blair, who had a cosmetics line that was well known in the region. Ginger swore by this neck exercise. When she passed away at a ripe old age, she still looked 50. Now Stanley is a great-grandfather, but he has the jawline and neck of a 40-year-old. He's the one who shared this magical exercise with me. So, let's thank both Stanley and Ginger!

Note: If you have a temporomandibular disorder (TMD) or another jaw-related problem, please check with your doctor to make sure it's okay for you to perform this exercise.

CAMP LESSON
YOUR FACE IS LIKE A THROW PILLOW

During each week of Beauty Camp, I'll present a lesson that will not only enhance what you've been learning in the week's activities but also pave the way for future camp sessions. In this first lesson, I want to talk about how and why our faces change as we get older.

If campers come to understand a few simple things about the structure and composition of skin, they'll be able to take two vitally important steps toward looking their best. First, they will understand how certain ingredients and molecules interact with skin cells and truly can reverse the effects of aging. Second, they will learn what I feel is one of the most important lessons for all Beauty Campers: how to read the ingredient list of a skin-care product.

Beauty Camp is about not taking claims on faith or buying into trends that don't have any basis in science. I am always curious about and open to anecdotal evidence; I listen carefully to the results that my patients—as well as my family and friends—report after using certain products. But at the end of the day, we must base our skin-care decisions on empirical realities, not on hopes and dreams and promises. When we stray from science, we are defenseless against false claims and at risk for becoming victims of marketing hype. That's why the products and procedures recommended throughout this book are, first and foremost, the fruits of scientific research.

Anatomy of Your Facial Skin

For purposes of this lesson, I want you to imagine a throw pillow. It is stuffed with foam, not down or feathers, and encased in soft, plush velour. When you first brought home your pillow, it may have been covered with a thin, almost invisible plastic wrap. This helped protect the pillow, keeping it smooth and firm.

Over the years, as you squish and crumple your pillow hundreds of times, its appearance gradually changes. The velour cover wears out; the color fades. The stuffing starts to crumble, so the pillow loses its shape. It isn't the pillow it once was.

Your facial skin is rather like that throw pillow. For example, on the surface is a layer of dead skin cells called the *stratum corneum*. Just as the plastic wrap on your pillow would get dirty and dingy if you left it in place, the stratum corneum becomes rough and dull as you get older.

If you were to examine the stratum corneum under a microscope, you'd see that it has a brick-and-mortar structure. The bricks are the dead skin cells, and the mortar is skin lipids—

large molecules that sit on the surface of the skin to hold in moisture and keep it soft and smooth. But two unfortunate things happen with age: The dead cells get thicker and thicker, while the moisture-trapping lipids diminish. These two factors combine to give skin a rough texture and lackluster appearance.

Directly beneath the exterior wrapping of the stratum corneum is the living *epidermis*. There is a characteristic wavy, undulating pattern to the cells in this layer. The uppermost cells are known as *squamous* cells; the lowermost are referred to as *basal* cells because of their position at the base of the epidermis.

Younger skin has a thick, hearty epidermis, like the plush velour cover of that new pillow. As the skin ages—as early as our twenties, especially in sun-exposed areas like the face, neck, and chest—this layer of living skin cells becomes smaller and flatter, much as velour wears out with use.

Please don't feel discouraged! All kinds of products, including exfoliants, moisturizers, and lipid replacements, can plump up a thinning epidermis. In fact, you'll see significant improvement in the appearance of your skin with simple topical applications of the right ingredients.

The Dermis: Where Trouble Begins

Right beneath the epidermis is another layer called the *dermis*. Whereas the epidermis consists primarily of cells, the dermis is mostly fluid and fibers. The two main fibers are *collagen* and *elastin*. (My guess is that you've heard these words before.)

In young skin, the dermis has loads of collagen and elastin. The fibers are very well organized; they act as good filler substances for the skin, so the surface stays smooth and plump. Older skin has less collagen and elastin, and the quality of the fibers isn't as good. They clump and degrade, much as a pillow's foam stuffing crumbles over time. Because of this deterioration, the fibers don't provide the fill and support that they do in young skin.

In the simplest terms, a wrinkle is an area of the skin in which the fibrous content of the dermis has declined, causing what looks to the naked eye like a groove. And because the skin lacks a strong, fibrous framework, it begins to sag. The scientific term for the deterioration of the fibers is *solar elastosis*, alluding to the fact that the damage is sun induced. When this damage becomes very advanced, it is reminiscent of a pillow losing its shape because the stuffing has broken down so significantly.

So the dermis is where it's all happening in terms of wrinkles and grooves, and it shows as well the more dramatic effects of time and sun exposure. But there's something else you need to know about this layer. In addition to the fibrous network of collagen and elastin, the dermis contains a chemical called *hyaluronic acid*. In younger skin, a healthy amount of hyaluronic (pronounced holl-yur-ON-ic) acid acts as a sponge, holding water in place to help hydrate the skin. In this way, it keeps skin looking plump and full while reducing any creases or sagging. The only problem is, hyaluronic acid content also diminishes as we get older.

What Skin-Care Products Can Do for You

By now you may be feeling as though you're fighting a losing battle against time, no matter what your current age. Rest assured, you have every reason to remain hopeful! In the weeks ahead, you'll discover skin-care ingredients and products that really can help repair and prevent skin damage. My intention in explaining the structure of the skin and how aging affects it is to help you better understand how particular products are meant to work.

For now, all you need to remember are the three substances in the dermis that go missing or go haywire over time: collagen, elastin, and hyaluronic acid. Recite them, highlight them, write them in the margin, because in Week #2 of Beauty Camp, when we begin to build a skin-care regimen just for you, we will be reading the ingredient labels on popular antiaging skincare products. The primary ingredients attempt to do one or more of the following:

1. Reduce the thickness of the stratum corneum (the dead skin-cell layer)
2. Build the epidermis (the living cell layer)
3. Improve collagen
4. Improve elastin
5. Improve hyaluronic acid
6. Improve the water content of the skin

Week #1 Review

- *Examine your Orientation photos.*
- *Get 30 minutes more sleep each night.*
- *Use 400-thread-count, all-cotton pillowcases.*
- *Wash those pillowcases (and anything else that will touch your face) in All Free Clear laundry detergent.*
- *Practice your facial exercises each day.*

Week #2

Basic Training
This week's agenda:
Learning which ingredients really work—and
how to find them on any product label

All of us have met at least one woman who swears by some old-fashioned or obscure wrinkle remedy. Certainly, all kinds of ingredients and products have promised to help reduce the appearance of facial lines. I'm sure some of them work in some way; otherwise, they would not have remained on the market for as many years as they have.

For instance, lots of my older patients are big fans of cold creams, and are almost sentimentally attached to them. I've studied the labels of these products. They tend to be concoctions of mineral oil, water, and beeswax—none of which has been proven to prevent or reduce wrinkles. In other words, they aren't able to do any of the things that we discussed in Week #1: reducing the thickness of the stratum corneum; building the epidermal cell layer; improving collagen, elastin, or hyaluronic acid; or increasing the water content of the skin.

From a physician's perspective, I don't believe that cold creams can undo wrinkling. What, then, do I say about my

80-year-old patient with lovely skin that she attributes to the faithful use of cold cream? I am reminded of the adage "If it ain't broke, don't fix it."

Some women do indeed appear to be getting good results from a product that has no scientific basis for working. One possible explanation is that a cold cream somehow creates a barrier on the surface of the skin, providing protection—even to a modest degree—from the elements. Another explanation: Women who are in their eighties now did not spend their youths stretched out on beach towels and rotating in the sun like rotisserie chickens.

Back in the 1920s, when today's 80-year-olds were in their teens, there was a cultural and class bias against having a tan. Tans were the domain of farmers and laborers, who spent most of their waking hours toiling in the sun. Women were discouraged from participating in outdoor or beach-oriented recreation. If they went outside, they wore hats and covered up their skin. I probably don't need to point out that in those days, sunlamps (popular in the 1960s and 1970s) and tanning parlors didn't exist, either.

Modern dermatologists blame sun exposure before age 18 for the vast majority of *photoaging*, the medical term for the changes that occur in sun-damaged skin over time. These changes include, but are not limited to, uneven pigment and brown spots, blotching, sagging, wrinkles, and easily bruised and fragile skin.

But wait a second. You didn't come to Beauty Camp just to hear that most of your photoaging took place before you even reached your twenties! You came for remedies—and I have lots of them. I am determined to convince even the most skeptical

Beauty Campers that paying some attention to the ingredients in skin-care products and putting together a new daily regimen will work wonders for the health and appearance of their skin.

But before we even begin thinking about shopping for new products, we need to take a tour of your own inventory. Remember the big box that I asked you to bring to camp? You may want to grab it before you read on.

CAMP ACTIVITY #1
YOUR BOX OF STUFF

With your box in hand, go through your house and collect all the skin-care products that belong to you—even if you've never used them. Look under your bathroom sink and in your medicine cabinet, on your vanity and in your purse, and in every other place that you might have stashed that long-forgotten kiwi-strawberry-lime peel-off mask. Track down every cream, lotion, and oil; every cleanser, toner, and moisturizer; every tonic, gel, and medicated pad. That's right: all those bottles and tubes and jars!

While you're at it, you may as well gather up all of your cosmetics—including those 10 tubes of lipstick that are the exact same color but go by different names—and your hair-care products, too. We'll be getting to them later, in Week #5.

Your next task should be a bit like cleaning out your closet. If you haven't used a certain product in a couple of years, consider tossing it right here and now, unless you genuinely believe that you might try it once you understand what it does and how. Use your best judgment.

Even after you throw away the ancients, your box could be

so full that you barely can carry it. Maybe you feel a little sheepish when you look at it. You can't fathom why you bought all that stuff or what you were thinking at the time. Do you really need five kinds of moisturizer and so many different cleansers? Some of the items may come from the drugstore, others from a department store; perhaps even a few are from your dermatologist. It's hard not to remember that the eye creams never rescued you from the fine lines, as they promised, and that the lip plumpers actually irritated your skin or made it flake.

Your fellow Beauty Campers may marvel at all of your stuff. Some may shake their heads. But look inside their boxes at their bottles and tubes and jars. They'll feel a little sheepish, too.

Dollars and Sense

Now comes the hard part. Add up what you've spent on skin-care products over the past year. Be honest—and don't forget to include everything that you used up before coming to Beauty Camp.

If you're among a group of campers, ask everyone to write their totals on slips of paper, then share them. Who spent the most? Who looks the best? That's the funny part: Money can buy you lots of expensive promises, but it won't necessarily buy you a face with fewer Uninvited Elements (UEs).

Think about what those dollars might have done for you. They could have been spent on a better hairstyle or some stylish new clothes. They might have gotten you a series of glycolic peels at a doctor's office. They could have been deposited in your child's or grandchild's college fund.

I say these things not to be mean, just honest. My hope is

that by the time you leave Beauty Camp, you'll have all the necessary information and tools to be a smart, savvy skin-care consumer.

So many of us buy skin-care products based on compelling ads in magazines or the recommendation of the lovely department-store salesperson who works on commission. We take the products home, not really sure what they're supposed to do other than make us look attractive and youthful and wonderful—in some vague, nondescript way. We read the directions; maybe we follow them, maybe we don't.

A week goes by; do we look better? It's hard to tell. Another few weeks go by. We search our faces, looking for signs of improvement. We don't notice any difference. Perhaps tellingly, nobody else seems to notice a difference, either.

What Works for You?

Part of the problem is that we never know exactly what to expect from a skin-care product. The promises and claims on the label—things like "antiaging," "antiwrinkle," and "anti-acne"—are there because a certain ingredient has been found to produce those effects *in most people*. But to get a good sense of whether a product might work for us, we need to consider all of its ingredients and their respective amounts. (As a rule of thumb, skin-care preparations list their ingredients in descending order of concentration.)

This is why it's so important to not choose skin-care products based on the appeal of a marketing campaign or even a particular brand name. It's the ingredients in the product, not the promises on the packaging, that will improve or eliminate your UEs. You'll need to do some experimenting to find the ingredients that work best for you. (Don't worry—I'm here to guide you!)

Another problem is that we tend to buy our skin-care products separately and often on impulse. We think of the various items as functioning independently of each other, instead of considering how each one fits into an overall skin-care regimen.

It reminds me of something that happened on a recent trip to Florence, Italy. One day, as my husband and I browsed the local shops, I spotted a pair of brown suede pumps with adorable (and I do mean adorable) big, bright orange bows. I had to try them on. As I admired the shoes in the mirror, my husband remarked that though they were cute, they wouldn't go with much of anything in my wardrobe. I bought them anyway. On the rare occasions when I wear all brown or all white, they're great. For the most part, though, they sit in my closet. In retrospect, they probably weren't the smartest buy.

The same principle should apply when purchasing skin-care products. They shouldn't just take up space in our cabinets. They should be a good match for our skin, as well as for the other products in our skin-care regimens.

In my practice, so many of my female patients have told me that they love a particular alpha hydroxy acid (AHA) or retinoid, but they can't use it anymore because it irritates their skin too much. In most cases, I just tweak their regimens by adding a botanical cleanser and/or a lipid lotion. Then they're able to continue using the AHA or retinoid without problem—and they see really great improvement in their skin.

In a way, customizing a skin-care regimen is like preparing a favorite recipe: You need just the right combination of products in just the right proportions to achieve the expected results.

CAMP ACTIVITY #2
WHITTLING DOWN YOUR BOX OF STUFF

Now for your next task: I want you to go through the products that you've collected and separate them into three different piles. We'll call them the Not-Sures, the Discards, and the Essentials.

The Not-Sures: These are the products that you bought, but you don't know if they are doing anything. You might try them once in a while, but you haven't really committed to testing them. We all have too many of these!

This pile also is for the products that you're not sure you want to continue using for other reasons. Maybe a friend or your dermatologist recommended them. Perhaps they irritated your skin or were too drying when you first tried them. (Some effective antiaging products can be irritating and cause dry patches.)

Hold on to this pile. Armed with the knowledge that you'll gain a bit later in this week of Beauty Camp, you may have new insights into how these products are supposed to work and how you might use them for better results—or whether they're worth using at all. The truth is, it's quite possible that you already own all the necessary products to put together a terrific daily skin-care regimen, but you haven't been using them as effectively or as regularly as you should.

The Discards: These are products that you just don't like, no matter what. You might have bought them in a weak moment at a salon or day spa, and they cost so much that you couldn't bear to throw them out. But they aren't for you. Maybe you can't stand how a product smells or how heavy or sticky it is.

Part of putting together your ideal skin-care regimen is

finding products that you really want to use. But don't toss your discards in the trash just yet. It will be fun to study their labels. And if they contain some effective ingredients, think for a second: Could they help another Beauty Camper or a friend? You may not like a product, but it could be perfect for someone else.

The Essentials: I call these Essentials, even though I know that most women don't adhere to a strict daily or weekly skin-care regimen. They're the products that you use on a regular basis or would pack for a weekend getaway.

For most women, this pile will include a facial cleanser, a moisturizer or cream, and maybe an eye treatment with a special ingredient that claims to radically improve crow's-feet or dark circles. You might add some kind of exfoliating scrub or mask. Of course, there's a favorite shampoo and conditioner, and possibly a hair spray, gel, or mousse.

If you intend to continue using these products, I strongly urge you to find their ingredient lists. They should be right on the product labels or packaging. Another option is to check online at the manufacturer's Web site. If that fails, go back to where you purchased the product and spend a few minutes jotting down the ingredients as they appear on the box.

The more you like—and swear by—these products, the more I hope you'll consider sharing samples of them with your fellow Beauty Campers.

What Kind of Camper Are You?

Your piles of skin-care products can be revealing. For example, let's take a look at your Essentials. Are the products fairly new? Some women love to experiment with their routines.

The Beauty Camp Exchange

Swapping and sharing is a way of life at Beauty Camp, just as it was at summer camp when you were a girl. So why not start now? If you have a product that your fellow campers are dying to try, perhaps you could pass out small samples (a week's worth) in plastic travel jars or bottles. They're available in most drugstores, and they're great for sharing. Likewise, beauty supply stores carry disposable applicators, like the ones at cosmetics counters. They might work well for a single testing of a product like a mask or glycolic gel at a camp meeting.

As a mother with three daughters, I'm a diehard fan of sharing products. There's so much upside in terms of how much money you can save—and how many mistakes you can avoid. However, there are a few caveats for sharing safely and smartly.

- If you can't remember how long ago you bought a product but it seems to have been around for a while, be wary of using it yourself, much less sharing it. The preservatives in most products break down after 2 years. If a product is less than 2 years old, you probably can

They don't have much self-control while shopping at cosmetics counters or in beauty boutiques—and as a result, they're likely to end up with a groaning pile of Essentials that consists mostly of the very latest must-haves. Does this sound familiar? Then you might be the kind of Beauty Camper who loves to buy proceed without any precautions. Anything older is best discarded.

- When using a nonprescription topical preparation that was purchased at a dermatologist's office, such as a cleanser or moisturizing cream, be sure to pay close attention to the directions for application. These products tend to have higher concentrations of active ingredients than their commercially available counterparts. Therefore, they should be used only as directed. Prescription preparations never should be shared.

- If a product contains an acid, like glycolic, carefully read the label and follow the directions provided by the manufacturer. Be especially cautious with high-strength formulations. Do not try them if you have sensitive skin, serious skin (topical) allergies, fever blisters or cold sores, sunburn, a history of eczema, or infection-prone skin.

- Do not share products with a Beauty Camper who has a cold sore, a cold, or even the sniffles. There may be germs lurking in any jar of cream that she puts her fingers into.

products but doesn't have a great deal of discipline and follow-through in using them.

Another type of camper is more cautious by nature and less inclined to change her skin-care routine. This woman might have the opposite problem: no new products but lots of dedication. If this sounds like you, there may be one relatively new product in your pile of Essentials. The rest are items that you've been using for many, many years. You might swear by them or feel some sort of attachment to them because they've been in your repertoire for so long.

I'm not saying that a new product is better than what you are currently using. You may have everything you need already. But if you examined your Orientation photos and determined that your nasolabial folds (the heavy grooves running from the corners of your nose to the edges of your mouth) are getting more noticeable, your crow's-feet are out of control, or your lip lines and age spots are multiplying, then you might want to at least try something new. In recent years, there have been some truly remarkable advances in skin-care products. The formulations just keep getting better—more effective and less irritating.

In other words, if you aren't completely happy with how you look in your Orientation photos, then I suspect that at least some of your Essentials aren't the best products for you. Maybe they aren't good enough or strong enough, or—as I so often see in my practice—maybe they are *too* strong and are overworking your tired skin. Or it could be that you have all the right products, but you aren't using them to their greatest advantage.

I am not suggesting that you run out and invest in an entirely new skin-care regimen. You might need to buy only one or two new items—and be more intelligent and diligent in using the rest.

No matter which type of Beauty Camper you are, I want you to hang on to your Essentials for now. Continue using them as we carefully transition to a new and better skin-care regimen.

What to Expect from a Skin-Care Product

In general, every single product that you put on your face with the intent of improving your skin should be proven effective in at least one of the six areas that I mentioned earlier: reducing the thickness of the stratum corneum; building the epidermal cell layer; improving collagen, elastin, or hyaluronic acid; or increasing the water content of the skin. Now I'm going to reword and expand this list, so you know exactly—in plain language—what you should expect.

No matter where you purchase a skin-care product—at the corner drugstore, in an upscale department store, by mail order, online, or in a dermatologist's office—it should do at least one of the following:

- Lessen lines
- Lift sagging contours
- Balance skin tone
- Reduce redness
- Clear and minimize pores
- Hydrate inside and out
- Eliminate scales and flakes
- Lighten dark shadows around the eyes
- Provide sun protection

If you are currently using a product that doesn't effectively do any of these things—and I am talking about producing significant, noticeable improvement in your skin—then it's time to face facts and move on. If you are currently using a product that you like, but you aren't sure what it contains or whether it's really making a difference, then it's time to do some research. Every ingredient in a product is there for a reason. Before you apply the product to your face, you should know what that reason is.

SCARY CAMP STORY:
DIANA'S $800 DILEMMA

Diana (not her real name) is a 66-year-old woman who comes to my office once a year so that I can check her skin for cancers. During one particular visit, Diana told my nurse that she had two new spots on her chest that I needed to examine. She also wanted me to check all of her moles to be sure I didn't see any suspicious changes.

When I walked into the exam room and apologized for running late, Diana was as sweet as usual. She showed me the knitting that she'd brought with her. I checked the new spots on her chest; they were precancerous, so I treated them with liquid nitrogen. Afterward, I checked the rest of her skin, performing what a dermatologist would call a total body exam. I reassured her that all her moles and freckles, including the facial lesions, were nothing to worry about.

Diana did tend to have a red flush to her skin. Since she never expressed concern about it or asked for my advice, I didn't want to mention it, either. It could make her feel self-conscious. But this visit, when we were done with the rest of the exam, it was Diana who prompted a new focus on her face. She let out a small, slightly embarrassed giggle.

"Dr. Ciraldo," she said, "I saw a doctor on TV recently. He was talking about how you could make your skin younger and prettier. He even has a book out."

"Oh, did you buy the book?" I asked.

"More than that," Diana offered. "I went out and bought his products."

None of this seemed very troublesome to me. So I let Diana continue. "The problem is, the products were pretty expensive," she said. "I spent $800 in one day, and I really don't see that they've done anything for me. I think I need your opinion."

At this point, I proceeded with a few questions. What did Diana want to change about her face? Her complaints: dryness, redness, fine lines, and lackluster skin.

I explained that she probably would see pretty significant improvement in just a week or two if she were to stop all the products she had been using and start the following regimen.

1. Morning and night, wash her face with Plexlon, a sulfa-based prescription cleanser.

2. Mornings only, apply a zinc-based SPF 30-plus sunblock with the antiwrinkle ingredients Elhibin and Colhibin. These are known to prevent the breakdown of elastin and collagen fibers in the dermis.

Before Diana left my office, I took her photo. I also asked if she would return in a week for follow-up and a comparison shot.

The difference between her before-and-after photos is remarkable. There's red-faced Diana on the day that she asked me about her "$800 dilemma." And there she is 1 week later, after using my suggested skin-care regimen. The texture of her skin is noticeably smoother and the redness is much improved. Diana was very pleased with the results. The prescription cleanser cost her about $60 and the sunblock about $30—a fraction of what she had spent on all those products that left her looking less than her best.

Like so many of us, Diana had bought into the message that she could improve her appearance if she followed a one-size-fits-all skin-care "system." She paid a hefty price, both in dollars and in the appearance of her skin. Fortunately for her, the damage was correctable.

The point is, there isn't one skin-care solution for everyone. Each face presents its own dilemmas and mysteries. Diana's new regimen might not work for someone else—but her $800 bag of stuff just might. Our faces are different because our skin is different. So our skin-care regimens need to be different, too.

CAMP ACTIVITY #3
LOOKING AT YOUR LABELS

From your pile of Essentials or Not-Sures, choose a product that you want to investigate. Like most skin-care products, this one should have two labels. On the front label, you'll see a brand name, a product name, and something called an action name, which reveals what the manufacturer says the product can do.

The information on the back label varies from one product to the next, depending on the overall packaging. If the product comes without a box, the back label should provide the directions as well as the ingredients. If the product has a box, the ingredients probably are listed on the outside of the box—which most of us throw away once we start using the product. But it's the ingredients that we must pay attention to.

For some products, the ingredient lists are pretty simple—just a handful of items at most. Other lists seem to barely fit on their labels. If you're daunted by the small print, grab a magnifying glass!

What's In a(n Action) Name?

Let's go back to the front label. Does the product really do what the action name says? Yes—to a degree.

The cosmetics industry enjoys a self-policing safety panel. Manufacturers adhere to a code of ethics governing the claims they make. As long as the FDA doesn't get any troublesome complaints, it doesn't intervene. This is great for the cosmetics industry—but not so great for the consumer.

For the most part, the claims state that a product will "improve the appearance" of some Uninvited Element—whether it's wrinkles, pores, acne, or something else. The product won't promise to change the UE. The FDA doesn't check whether the product lives up to the claim. It only monitors the language of the claim—and not very closely, at that.

For the average consumer, these are very hazy distinctions—perhaps just a game of semantics. But I predict that they will become a point of contention in the not-too-distant future. Some manufacturers are performing laboratory studies in which biopsies show increased collagen in the skin after the use of certain ingredients—a sign that a true structural change has taken place. It isn't only about appearance anymore. Skin with more collagen really has fewer wrinkles.

Decoding the Ingredient List

Let's return to the back label and to the ingredient list in particular. It's important to know not only which ingredients are in the product, but also how much of each one. Many ingredients are effective only if they are present in a certain strength.

Take glycolic acid as an example. You'll come across this ingredient virtually everywhere that skin-care products are sold. In doctors' offices, it is offered in "physician-strength" formulations; in department stores, salons, and day spas—as well as online—it's available in so-called neutralized or buffered forms.

What is glycolic acid? Technically, it is the acid of sugarcane. As such, it often is marketed as a "natural" rejuvenator. If truth be told, the most common source of glycolic acid is the laboratory rather than sugarcane—but that isn't meant to diminish its value. Glycolic acid is one of the most effective ingredients in today's skin-rejuvenation business. It reduces the stratum corneum, the dead skin-cell layer. It builds the thickness of the epidermis, the living cell layer. It also increases collagen, elastin, and hyaluonic acid and improves skin hydration.

Most Beauty Campers probably will want some kind of glycolic acid product in their daily skin-care regimens. But not all glycolic acids are created equal. This is why you'll need to learn the rules for reading an ingredient list—and to not take for granted the claim on the front of a jar, tube, or bottle. A reasonably strong glycolic acid solution is necessary for a product to be effective. Otherwise, there's little point in using it at all.

I once saw an ad campaign in which a major skin-care company was pitching a 10 percent glycolic acid formula for under $10. This amazed me. Ten percent is a terrific strength, but I'd never seen such a product for under $25 or $30. Then I figured it out: The so-called 10 percent solutions aren't equal, either.

Many dermatologists, including me, dispense pure glycolic acid. This means that the acid hasn't been neutralized in any way. The product is very acidic, with a pH of about 3.5. (The pH level is a measurement of acidity; the stronger the glycolic acid solution, the lower the pH level.) But only a doctor's office or Web site can sell such strong formulations. This protects consumers from misuse that could cause irritation and a rash.

All the glycolic acid products that you'll see in drugstores and department stores are gentler than physician-strength formulations, with pH levels closer to the pH balance of the skin—around 6. The higher the pH, the less stinging and redness you'll experience. The results will be a little less dramatic with these products, compared with those of a physician-strength formulation. I'm not saying that the commercially available products can't do the trick. They simply are not as strong and therefore take longer to bring about noticeable improvement.

So when you see a label that mentions the percentage of glycolic acid in the product, be aware that how you interpret that percentage depends on the marketplace. Any product that is sold in a drugstore or department store as a "10 percent formula" is not 10 percent pure, undiluted glycolic acid. Rather, the formula contained 10 percent acid before being neutralized to meet product safety standards.

The more useful and accurate way to describe the strength of a solution is to specify the amount of "free" or "available" glycolic acid once the product has been neutralized. Because consumers may experience considerable irritation and peeling with a product containing 10 percent pure glycolic acid, most mass-marketed formulations have been diluted so that the free or available acid is in the range of 2 to 3 percent (even when the label says 10 percent). The point is, the percentage on the product label may not reflect the actual amount of glycolic acid that you're applying to your skin.

One of my patients learned this lesson the hard way. She

arrived at my office with a small bottle of a 50 percent glycolic acid peel that she'd purchased for $170 at the cosmetics counter of a major department store. Once she started using the product, she was very surprised to discover that it didn't tingle nearly as much as other peels that she had purchased in doctors' offices. She asked for my analysis—and she wasn't too happy when I explained that the amount of actual free glycolic acid in the bottle was less than the 10 percent she'd been getting in physician-strength formulations.

What you need to remember is this: Nonneutralized physician-strength formulations generally are several times more concentrated than their commercially available counterparts are.

Learning to Read Labels

To help you get the hang of deciphering labels, let's examine two products together. For this exercise, I've selected two cleansers from the Neutrogena line. This is a longtime favorite brand of dermatologists, so these products could be promising.

For product #1, here's what appears on the front label.

Product name: Neutrogena Healthy Skin Anti-Wrinkle Anti-Blemish Cleanser

Action name: "For Clear, Smooth Skin"

Other actions: Salicylic acid treats and helps prevent blemishes

Size: 5.1-ounce tube

Now let's take a look at the back label. This is where it gets really interesting.

Active ingredient: 0.5% salicylic acid

Inactive ingredients: Water, sodium methyl cocoyl taurate, cocamidopropyl betaine, sodium cocoampho-acetate, glycol distearate, glycolic acid, sodium lactate, cocamidopropyl PG-dimonium chloride phosphate, polyquaternium-11, disodium EDTA, fragrance

You'll notice that this label identifies two categories of ingredients: active and inactive. If an ingredient is "active," then the product is considered an over-the-counter drug with a very specific purpose. The manufacturer is required to disclose the percentage (or strength) of each active ingredient. Usually these products are sunscreens or, as is the case here, acne treatments.

This particular Neutrogena cleanser has only one active ingredient: salicylic acid, in 0.5 percent strength. Salicylic acid is one of my favorite pore-clearing and exfoliating ingredients. It's terrific as a cleanser. It is also proven to fight acne—thus the antiblemish claim on the front label.

Pretty straightforward, right? It is—until we turn our attention to the inactive ingredients. This is where reading labels can get murky. The inactive ingredient list on our cleanser is rather typical of skin-care products—lots of exotic-sounding chemicals but no percentages, so you can't be sure of the amounts or strengths. As a dermatologist who has been formulating skin-care products for myself and other physicians for 15 years, I can give you some idea of what this label is telling you.

As I mentioned earlier, all ingredients appear in descending order of concentration—which means this Neutrogena cleanser is mostly water. There's nothing wrong with that. Water is simply the medium, or the liquid, the manufacturer chose to use to deliver the salicylic acid and other good things to your skin.

The second ingredient, sodium methyl cocoyl taurate, also goes by the name ox bile. It's a fairly common emulsifier and yes, it is made from the fresh bile of castrated bulls, as its name suggests. It's totally safe for your skin, but the bull probably didn't enjoy his part in the process. So if you don't like the idea of animal-derived ingredients or prefer products that say "No Animal Testing," then you may want to steer clear of this product.

Next, we see something called cocamidopropyl betaine. Perhaps best known as an ingredient in eye-makeup removers, it is derived from a mixture of coconut oil and beets.

The fourth ingredient in the list, sodium cocoamphoacetate, is a surfactant. It allows the water in the cleanser to spread out and penetrate more easily.

Then comes glycol distearate, another surfactant. It contains glycerin and stearic acid, a fatty, almost buttery substance that imparts a creamy consistency to products like hand creams.

After the water and the surfactant ingredients, we finally get to some substance: glycolic acid and sodium lactate. Both are alpha hydroxy acids, which are very good in a skin-care product. They should provide some additional pore-clearing, antiacne, and antiwrinkle effects.

Whenever you see an "acid" in an ingredient list, it means that the ingredient has not been diluted or buffered. The glycolic in our cleanser is called an acid, which tells you that it is in pure acid form. This is important information because, as I've said before, glycolic acid may be less effective when it has been neutralized. By comparison, sodium lactate is lactic acid (derived from milk) that has been buffered with sodium hydroxide to make it less irritating—and, some would argue, less effective.

Continuing with our list, the next ingredient is cocamido-propyl PG-dimonium chloride phosphate, a derivative of coconut oil that's used as a lathering agent. Polyquaternium-11, a derivative of ammonium chloride, is a common ingredient in deodorants. If you are sensitive to deodorants, you may not want to use skin-care products that have a lot of polyquaternium-11 in them.

Disodium EDTA acts like a water softener. No matter how hard the water you're using, you will be left with smoother skin when you cleanse with this product.

Last in the list is fragrance. Finally, something self-explanatory!

Now that we've gone through all the inactive ingredients, let's return to glycolic acid and sodium lactate and their locations in the list. They're so far down—right before the preservatives, dyes, and fragrance—that they must be present in very small concentrations.

Remember, both glycolic acid and lactic acid are AHAs. Buying a good AHA product is like buying real estate: It all comes down to location, location, location. Since both acids fall just before the preservatives on this label, you can bet that the product contains no more than 1 percent of either ingredient.

Is this strong enough? No. To see a noticeable improvement from AHAs, you need a product with at least 5 percent acid, even if the 5 percent is from all the acid ingredients combined.

If the ingredient you're looking for appears after the fragrance on the label, you're really in dire shape. Usually fragrance is just 0.25 to 0.5 percent of a solution.

Now let's compare this Neutrogena cleanser with another—also from the Neutrogena line—that's touted to help acne. From the front label:

Product name: Oil-Free Acne Wash, 60 Second Mask Scrub

Action name: "2-in-1 Mask Scrub Effectively Clears Breakouts"

Size: 6-ounce tub

And from the back label:

Active Ingredient: 1% salicylic acid

Inactive Ingredients: Water, glycerin, kaolin, bentonite, sodium methyl cocoyl taurate, titanium dioxide, polyethylene, microcrystalline wax, trideceth 9, PEG-5, ethylhexanoate, menthol, ferric ferrocyanide, xanthan gum, disodium EDTA, sodium citrate, citric acid, phenoxyethanol, fragrance

Right off the bat, this looks like a better buy. It contains twice as much salicylic acid as the first cleanser and therefore should be twice as effective. Any cleanser with 1 percent salicylic acid is going to help clear acne and minimize pores. It also will help improve dull-looking skin, as well as the appearance of wrinkles. (This product is a bargain pricewise, too—$6.99 for 6 ounces, versus $7.99 for 5.1 ounces of the first cleanser.) But let's look at the rest of the label.

There's water and then glycerin, which I love for its ability to trap water. This normalizes the water balance of the skin and improves the structure of the stratum corneum (the dead skin-cell layer).

Next in the list are kaolin and bentonite, two natural clays that can draw out skin impurities to clean pores and sweep dead skin cells from the surface. You'll remember sodium methyl cocoyl taurate from before, so I won't repeat the ox bile story here. It's followed (in order) by titanium dioxide, a whitener; polyethylene, an abrasive scrub agent; and microcrystalline wax, a thickener.

Trideceth 9 helps to maintain the acidity of the salicylic acid in the wash, while PEG-5 and ethylhexanoate help to dissolve the other ingredients. Menthol is cooling to the skin. Ferric ferrocyanide gives color to the product, and xanthum gum helps thicken it. Disodium EDTA is the softener we discussed earlier. The rest of the ingredients are preservatives and fragrance.

Here's my assessment: Even if you don't take into consideration the inactive ingredients, this looks like a good acne treatment and pore cleanser. You can tell by the strength of the salicylic acid. The only thing that would make me hesitate to recommend it is the fragrance. When I tested the product on my own face, I turned red and blotchy. So if you have sensitive skin, as I do, you might shy away from this product—and anything else with fragrance.

A Word about Fragrance

When you see fragrance among the ingredients on a product label, it most likely is artificial—like a perfume. This isn't a bad thing, unless you don't like the scent—or you're allergic to it. In fact, even if a product gets its scent from the natural oil of a fragrant flower, you may experience a reaction to it. Many people who are sensitive to strong smells find that they have just as much of a problem with botanically enhanced "natural" products as with artificial ones.

Tricks of the Label-Reading Trade

I know what you may be thinking: *I'm not a chemist. This label-reading stuff is too confusing.* But there are some tricks to make it easier—and to help you find products in strengths that will be most beneficial for your face.

Trick #1: As a rule of thumb, if an ingredient is one of the last five in the list on the product label (or one of the last 10 of a very long list), then you won't be getting enough of the ingredient to make a difference in your skin. The exceptions are the retenoids; they will always be less than 1 percent, and always appear last in the ingredients list.

Trick #2: Learn to recognize the names of common preservatives in skin-care products. By law, skin-care products must contain preservatives to keep the formulas stable. Usually the percentage is small—1 percent or less. So if an ingredient such as glycolic acid appears right before the preservatives, the product probably contains no more than 1 percent of that ingredient. Among the most common preservatives in skin-care products:

Caprylyl glycol

Citric acid

Diazolidinyl urea (germall 11)

DMDM hydantoin

Imidazolidinyl urea (germall 115)

Methylchloroisothiazolinone

Methylisothiazolinone

Parabens (sometimes called phenonip; also identified by the prefixes butyl, ethyl, isobutyl, methyl, and propyl)

Pentylene glycol

Phenoxyethanol

Sorbic acid

Quaternium-15

Trick #3: The Internet is an invaluable resource for tracking down information on the uses and effectiveness of a particular ingredient, as well as brand-name products that contain it. Sometimes you can buy just a small amount of an ingredient online, if it's something that you want to test on your skin.

One of my patients introduced me to www.truetest.com, which identifies 24 topical ingredients that commonly cause allergies. If you seem to be having a reaction to a particular skin-care product, I suggest visiting this Web site and checking the ingredient list of the product against the one on the site. If you identify an ingredient that may be causing trouble, please take the time to read more about it. You may want to avoid this and related ingredients when choosing products.

Trick #4: For shopping trips and exploratory missions, you may want to purchase one of the following references: *Milady's Skin Care and Cosmetic Ingredients Dictionary*, by Natalia Michalun; or *A Consumer's Dictionary of Cosmetic Ingredients*, by Ruth Winter. (If you're attending Beauty Camp in a group, perhaps everyone could chip in to buy one of these books to share.) Both are available in paperback and handy enough to carry in your purse or tote bag. Although these dictionaries will not inform you of the latest ingredients on the market, they will give you insights into the most frequently used ingredients in many skin-care lines.

CAMP LESSON
MY FAVORITE INGREDIENTS

Knowing the right ingredients is like knowing the right people: doors open; things happen. I have been formulating skin-care products for about 15 years now, and I can attest that the right ingredients in the right combinations can dramatically improve your skin's appearance. It is a fact.

A good marketing campaign will convince you to rely on a brand name. I want you to learn to trust an ingredient instead. In Week #3 of Beauty Camp, we will assemble a new daily skin-care regimen for you. Hopefully, you'll develop some new skin-care habits, too. But before you can assess your current inventory of products or add new ones to it, you need to learn about specific active ingredients—and, more important, find the right ones for you.

It isn't necessary to memorize the following list. Simply read through it once (or maybe twice), and you will be light-years ahead as a Beauty Camper and consumer. These are the ingredients that really can make things happen for your skin. I'll try to mention them as often as possible throughout the rest of the book. That way, you'll begin to recognize them almost automatically!

The ingredients appear in alphabetical order here. Some are followed by what's known as an INCI name. INCI stands for "international nomenclature cosmetic ingredient." Manufacturers may use the INCI names in product labels, so you should be aware of them.

When you see an asterisk (*) before a particular name, it means that I consider the ingredient a must-have for myself.

A Note for Moms-to-Be

If you are pregnant, be sure to consult your obstetrician or dermatologist for guidance on which skin-care products you can use—and which you should avoid. For example, retinoids are a definite no-no for moms-to-be. On the other hand, sunscreen is more important than ever; during pregnancy, your skin can become a veritable magnet for the sun.

Many other active ingredients in skin-care products have not been thoroughly tested on pregnant women. Ask your doctor for guidance.

You may want to include it in your daily regimen, too, if you aren't using it already.

Algae Peptides
(brand name: Apt; INCI name: water, butylene glycol, ahnfeltia concinna extract)

Peptides in skin-care products are quite the rage—and with good reason. These small molecules can penetrate the epidermis to reach the skin layer (the dermis) beneath.

Algae peptides have the advantage of producing rapid, visible changes—tightening and the appearance of firming. I have been fascinated with these peptides since 1993, when I began incorporating them into a skin-care line that I make for myself and other physicians. Among their components is hydroxyproline, an unusual amino acid rarely found in the skin except within its own collagen.

When an algae peptide is applied to the skin, it is picked up by binding sites on the cells of the epidermis as well as the dermis. This seems to help explain the peptide's range of activities, which include increases in cell turnover and collagen synthesis. Using products with algae peptides can enhance the hydration, smoothness, elasticity, and fullness of the skin.

Aloe Vera

Years ago, one of my patients (hello, Bert!) gave me cuttings from his magnificent aloe vera plant. I have been taking advantage of the gooey juice inside the succulent leaves ever since, particularly when I burn myself while cooking. Many scientific studies demonstrate the effectiveness of aloe vera in soothing and reducing inflammation, healing wounds, and even increasing bloodflow.

With so many antiaging products being composed of various acids—which are irritants used in a controlled fashion to exfoliate and plump the skin—aloe vera has proven useful as a natural calming agent. When we spot it in the ingredient list of a product label, it's like seeing the name of a good friend.

*Alpha Hydroxy Acids

"Alpha hydroxy acids" is the chemical description of a group of ingredients that includes glycolic, lactic, and malic acids.

By far the most commonly used of the AHAs is glycolic acid. It is the smallest molecule of these acids and, therefore, it seems to penetrate best. Lactic acid also is an effective exfoliant but is not as popular, partly because glycolic is considered more effective. (I'll say much more about glycolic acid in just a bit.)

Antioxidants

(Including alpha lipoic acid; beta-carotene; coenzyme Q10; emblica; green tea; idebenone; panthenol; and topical vitamins A, C, and E)

When we say that an ingredient has "antioxidant activity," we meant that it protects against cellular oxidation. This is the breakdown that occurs when molecules known as free radicals form in the skin—the result of a variety of environmental insults, including sun exposure, pollution, smoking, and excessive alcohol consumption. Free radicals contribute to cellular aging and increase the risk of skin cancer, due to changes in the cellular nucleus. By neutralizing free radicals, antioxidants may prevent cellular aging and skin cancer.

Vitamin C is the granddaddy of antioxidant ingredients in skin-care products; we'll discuss it in further detail below. Among the best-studied of the topical antioxidants is green tea. Well-controlled trials involving laboratory animals have shown that topical application of green tea reduces not only inflammation but also tumors that can result from intense ultraviolet exposure.

The most heavily marketed of the antioxidant formulas contains idebenone, which is sold under the brand name Prevage—shorthand for "prevents aging." (Allergan, the manufacturer, is a huge pharmaceutical company that makes the prescription retinoid Tazorac, as well as Botox Cosmetic injections.)

Prevage launched with great fanfare, including a cover story in *W* magazine that described it as "the beauty cream with a waiting list." But disappointing sales prompted the manufacturer to team up with Elizabeth Arden and totally revamp its presentation of the product. The packaging changed from a

1-ounce plastic tube to a sleek, silver-toned pump bottle. What's more, distribution of the product moved from doctors' offices to department-store cosmetics counters.

Why didn't Prevage take off as expected? I certainly don't know the whole answer, but based on the feedback that I've gotten, it just didn't seem to deliver the fast results that Tazorac does.

Bentonite

This American white clay appears mostly in masks and acne treatments. Like other clays, such as kaolin, it can absorb oil and tighten the skin.

Benzoyl Peroxide

If you're familiar with Clearasil, Stridex, or Proactiv, then you know benzoyl peroxide. It's a tried-and-true acne treatment that clears and dries pores. It is also antibacterial and anti-inflammatory.

Unfortunately, about 10 percent of people are allergic to benzoyl peroxide and can develop skin irritation if they continue to use it—a tricky situation when treating acne, which causes redness to begin with. Because you can develop irritation even if you aren't allergic to benzoyl peroxide, I suggest taking a break from it every few months. If your old acne spots stay red despite treatment with benzoyl peroxide, try switching to another antiacne regimen, such as glycolic acid and salicylic acid.

My favorite prescription topical acne treatments, Duac gel and BenzaClin gel, combine benzoyl peroxide with topical antibiotics. These seem more effective than topical formulations of antibiotics alone. And because they clear the skin faster, they can be used for shorter periods of time and therefore tend to be less problematic.

*Botanicals

The botanicals include scores of plant-derived ingredients. Some you may readily recognize, like chamomile, echinacea, grape seed extract, and lavender. For people without fragrance sensitivities, just the scent of botanicals can be calming and soothing. Formulations with two or three botanicals can balance the sometimes harsh activities of other skin-care products, from shedding dead skin cells to enhancing skin texture. But if you have sensitive skin or a sensitive nose, then I'd steer clear of formulations with more than four botanicals—or particularly exotic ones.

Camphor
(INCI name: Cinnamomum camphora)

Camphor is a tightening ingredient. Like the clays (bentonite and kaolin) and even some botanicals (such as menthol and pumpkin), it is wonderful for short-term use but generally not meant to be left on the skin. You'll see camphor in masks and other wash-off skin-care products.

Chamomile
(INCI name: Matricaria chamomilla)

This daisylike flower is a popular ingredient in skin-care products. It imparts a calming effect with its gentle scent, as well as its healing properties.

*Colhibin

(INCI name: hydrolyzed rice peptides)

Colhibin is a plant-derived peptide that works by inhibiting collagenases, the enzymes that break down collagen. Studies have shown that as little as 2 percent Colhibin in a skin-care formulation can produce a 50 percent reduction in the activity of collagenases. In this way, Colhibin helps protect collagen against the effects of aging, sun exposure, and other environmental stresses. Even sun exposure not significant enough to redden the skin (called *suberythema doses of ultraviolet radiation*) can break down collagen.

*Elhibin

(INCI name: soybean, orglycine soja, protein)

Another plant-derived peptide, Elhibin, works similarly to Colhibin, except Elhibin's job is to protect against the deterioration of elastin—which, like collagen, provides structure to the skin—by blocking the enzyme elastase.

Irritation caused by sun exposure, environmental stresses, or ordinary dryness leads to the accumulation of white blood cells in the skin, which release large amounts of elastase. When uncontrolled, elastase affects the elastin fibers in all connective tissue—not only the skin but blood vessels, too. This in part explains the broken blood vessels that we see in chronically sun-exposed, sun-damaged skin.

The good news is that the body continues to produce elastin. By preventing its breakdown, Elhibin has the ability to replenish the skin, reduce irritation, and increase hydration.

*Eyeliss

(INCI name: water, glycerin, hesperidin methyl chalcone, stea-
reth-20, dipeptide-2, palmitoyl tetrapeptide-3)

Eyeliss is a trademarked ingredient that's found in a good number of new eye treatments on the market. Essentially, it's a con-
coction of peptides that, when applied topically, prevents the
capillaries in areas of very thin skin from leaking—which
means it can erase dark shadows or circles under the eyes.
Other substances in Eyeliss can restore elasticity and firmness
to the skin, as well as draw fluid from under the eyes to eliminate bags.

Glycerin

You'll most often find glycerin in cleansers and other wash-off
skin-care products. Although it has an amazing water-trapping
quality that normalizes water balance and restores structure to
the stratum corneum (the dead skin-cell layer), its slightly
gummy texture can leave the skin feeling sticky if it isn't
washed off. That said, I happen to like glycerin as an ingredient. If you're using a glycerin-containing leave-on product, just
apply it very sparingly, and you shouldn't have any problem.

*Glycolic Acid

(may appear on labels as ammonium or sodium glycolate)

We discussed glycolic acid a bit earlier in the chapter, but it's so
popular as an antiaging ingredient that we should revisit it
here. Its popularity is due in large part to its effectiveness—to
which most glycolic acid users will attest.

Studies conducted by Eugene Van Scott, MD, of the Tem-
ple University department of dermatology have proven glycolic

acid to be a very potent skin rejuvenator that begins to exfoliate almost immediately upon application. Because it is such a good exfoliant, some people worry that it might thin their skin. Rest assured, it isn't cause for concern.

Glycolic acid, like any exfoliant, will thin the stratum corneum. This is why people who use glycolic acid products notice a healthy new "glow" to their skin: The dead cells of the stratum corneum no longer obscure the living cells of the epidermis, so the surface of the skin looks more radiant. With continued treatments, the epidermis will thicken, further restoring the skin's appearance. Over time, the skin will manufacture new collagen, elastin, and hyaluronic acid, as well.

Some people report significant cosmetic improvement to the epidermal layer within days of beginning glycolic acid treatments. Changes to the dermal layer—like a reduction in the appearance of fine lines—usually take at least 2 weeks.

If your skin doesn't seem irritated by the glycolic acid products you've purchased at drugstores or department stores and you're hoping for more dramatic results, you might try a formulation sold under a dermatologist's label. Many of these higher-strength formulas can be purchased by phone or online and do not require an office visit. Make sure that the product you order has a lower pH level than the retail brand you've already tried. (As explained earlier, a lower pH level means the product is more acidic and stronger.)

The pH level is an independent factor influencing the effectiveness of a product. One study published in 1993 by Walter Smith, PhD, a well-respected independent cosmetic chemist, showed that a drop of 2 in the pH level correlated to an increase of 30 percent in cell turnover rate (one measurement of skin rejuvenation). So, if a dermatologist's formulation has a pH of

4 (generally, doctors' products are around 3.5) and a store brand has a pH of 6, you can expect about 30 percent better results from the dermatologist's formulation based solely on its more acidic nature.

For even more dramatic improvement in your skin's appearance, you might consider an in-office glycolic acid treatment, which will have a higher percentage of glycolic acid and a lower pH. For example, in-office glycolic acid peels, which are applied and then washed off, have pH levels closer to 1 to 2. So you can expect significant unclogging of pores and lessening of roughness and excess pigment buildup after some in-office glycolic acid treatments.

Hyaluronic Acid

(May appear on labels as sodium hyalurmate)

We've talked about hyaluronic acid as a chemical that occurs naturally in the dermis. You can also find it in skin-care products. It is what's known as a humectant, capable of holding 1,000 times its weight in water. I like to describe it as a sponge that plumps out the skin.

Interestingly, the molecules of topical hyaluronic acid are too large to travel to the dermis. It acts only on the epidermis, where it's an effective moisturizing ingredient. The molecules of glycolic acid are comparatively smaller, so they can reach the dermis—and once there, they help stimulate production of hyaluronic acid.

Therefore, if you want a moisturizing effect without the potential for irritation, I recommend hyaluronic acid. It will help remedy flaky skin and soften skin texture by increasing hydration. If you also want to fill in fine lines, then a product with glycolic acid would be your best bet. (Or use both, as I do.)

Hydroquinone

Hydroquinone (pronounced hydro-QUINN-own) is a chemical that prevents skin cells from making new pigment. It is a very effective bleaching ingredient—the best in any fade preparation—and works well as a treatment for age spots, brown dots, or masklike stains from pregancy or oral contraceptives. It also does a good job with certain kinds of dark under-eye circles.

Hydroquinone comes in a variety of formulations. If you are prone to acne, look for a solution, lotion, or gel rather than a heavy cream. Preparations containing at least 3 percent hydroquinone are available by prescription only, but the lower concentrations in over-the-counter products can be very effective when paired with glycolic acid. In my 25 years of dermatologic experience, I've found that for many people, this duo works as well as prescription-strength hydroquinone.

Kaolin

This is another good clay ingredient, usually found in masks and acne treatments. While bentonite is a white substance found in America, whitish yellow kaolin is Asian—mostly from China (hence its other name, China clay). Both clays have exceptional oil-absorbing abilities and can reduce shine when left on the skin for 20 minutes, then gently rinsed off.

*Lipids
(including ceramides, glycolipids, and sphingolipids)

Lipids are the natural, protective layer of fats that cover a newborn's skin. We lose this layer over time, for a variety of reasons. For example, all methods of exfoliation—which accelerate removal of the stratum corneum, the dead skin-cell layer—strip away lipids, as well. They also can become depleted by sun exposure or a dry environment—including the dryness that occurs when running a dehumidifier or air conditioner. Many of my patients have complained that their skin becomes noticeably drier and rougher when they use certain drugs, both topical preparations (like prescription retinoids) and pills (like cholesterol-lowering medications). Perhaps not surprisingly, aging takes a toll on lipids, too.

I recommend replacing these naturally occurring lipids with a topical product that contains them. They sit on the stratum corneum, where they protect the skin and keep it well hydrated and young looking.

In case you aren't familiar with lipids as a skin-care ingredient (most women aren't), I thought I'd provide a few leads on products that you may want to check out. A new line called CeraVe incorporates ceramides and cholesterol into a cleanser, cream, and lotion—each priced at about $1 an ounce. Look for it in drugstores. L'Oréal offers Nutrissime, with omega-ceramides. It's available in many drugstores and large supermarkets. And Elizabeth Arden has a very popular product, Ceramide, which you'll find in better department stores.

Microdermabrasion Particles

Usually these are aluminum oxide crystals; they feel like fine grains of sand on your face. I sometimes joke that trying these creams is like a day at the beach because they leave behind a sandy residue that must be rinsed thoroughly.

Dermatologists apply microdermabrasion particles with machines that buff (or *dermabrade*) the outer layer of skin—

whether to smooth out shallow acne scars, impart a glow to sallow skin, or lessen the appearance of fine lines. You can find microdermabrasion creams for home use as well.

Just one caveat: If you are very aggressive with a microderm-abrasion cream, your skin will turn red from it. At the first sign of redness, please stop using the cream immediately. Do not apply any AHAs or retinoids to your skin until the redness subsides.

Mineral Oil

I'm not sure how mineral oil came to have a reputation as *comedogenic* (or acne causing), but most studies now exonerate it as a pore clogger. This much-maligned ingredient really is harmless.

Minerals

Minerals have been credited with moisturizing and skin-firming properties for centuries. The Ahava brand, which is manufactured at the Dead Sea and laden with minerals, has introduced a Time Line product line for skin rejuvenation. Lancôme is offering its own calcium-laden line.

Mineral-based makeup, which is becoming quite popular, refracts light rays off the skin so that it looks almost flawless. Manufacturers claim that the makeup is so mild it can be left on overnight. I advise against this, as proper nighttime cleansing is essential for getting optimal results from your skin-care regimen.

*Neuropeptides

(including argireline [INCI name: acetyl hexapeptide-3], and GABA complex)

You might hear neuropeptides described as topical Botox because they act on the sort of facial lines and furrows that usually are treatable with Botox Cosmetic injections. Whereas the injections produce a paralytic effect by preventing nerves from releasing acetylcholine, a neurotransmitter that instructs muscles to contract, neuropeptides inhibit only the chemical. Therefore, the muscles can still contract but not as vigorously—and the effect is reversible.

For some people, neuropeptides can help lessen the appearance of dynamic lines. Of course, a product must have a certain concentration of neuropeptides to achieve results. So look for a product that mentions neuropeptides near the top of its ingredient list. Be forewarned: Some of these products are among the most highly priced in the entire skin-care industry. In studies, neuropeptides have produced at best a 50 percent reduction in certain dynamic lines. Then again, even injectable Botox can't guarantee 100 percent effectiveness.

I recommend neuropeptide products for areas where Botox isn't appropriate—usually around the eyes (closer to the eyes than crow's-feet), lips, and neck. Some women prefer to combine the two treatments for maximum effect. In fact, many younger women who certainly should not yet be considering Botox Cosmetic injections are getting good results with topical neuropeptides. My daughter Gina, who is 24, applies them faithfully twice a day. This makes sense to me, as long-term use could lessen the appearance of dynamic lines. (By the way, if you're curious about injectable Botox, we'll discuss it in much greater detail when we get to Beauty Camp Extra on page 207.)

*Oxygen Activators
(may appear on labels as yeast extract)

If I were to choose just one skin-care product to have with me on a deserted island, it would contain an oxygen activator. It's an antisag remedy that really works for me.

As we age, our cellular metabolism and the accompanying oxygen consumption decline, which is why our skin starts to sag. An oxygen activator somehow steps up cellular metabolism, akin to what exercise does for muscles. I have found, though, that the effect seems less dramatic for women who are already in their late sixties or older.

Panthenol

This ingredient is derived from vitamin B_5 (pantothenic acid)—which is exactly what it's converted to when applied to the skin. Panthenol acts as a humectant, trapping water to smooth the skin's surface. You'll find it not only in moisturizers (among other skin-care products) but also in the top-selling Pantene hair-care line.

Papaya

This tropical fruit contains the enzyme papain, which is used as a meat tenderizer. In skin-care formulations, papaya dissolves dead cells from the skin's surface as well as from pores. A papaya preparation works best if you massage it into skin and leave it on for some time before rinsing off.

*Peptides

Peptides are chains of amino acids. Cosmetic chemists differentiate between peptides that are beneficial to the skin and those that are not. When a peptide is proven in laboratory testing to improve the skin in some way, it is classified as an active peptide. Among these are algae peptides, Colhibin, Elhibin, Eyeliss, and neuropeptides—all of which we discussed earlier.

Some active peptides are antibacterial, while others either

bind to enzymes or inhibit enzymes that break down skin structure, as is the case with Colhibin and Elhibin. Still others function much like retinoids, stimulating collagen production and binding to retinoid receptors in the skin. In one study, more than 30 percent of people who used peptides saw immediate improvement in their skin, while another 5 percent saw improvement within several hours. Almost 70 percent of users reported tighter, firmer skin within 2 weeks.

Retinoids

(prescription: Avage, Differin, Retin-A, Retin-A Micro, Renova, Tazorac, tretinoin, Tri-Luma; nonprescription: retinol, an Ingredient In products marketed under many different brand names)

Retinoids are vitamin A derivatives that act as antioxidant, antipigment, and exfoliant agents. They also increase production of collagen and hyaluronic acid, which is how they help firm the skin.

Perhaps the best known of the retinoids is tretinoin, or Retin-A. Although the term *cosmeceutical* has been around since 1962, Retin-A was the first product to truly merit the classification by bridging the gap between a cosmetic and a pharmaceutical. Originally developed as a topical treatment for acne, it later was found to reduce wrinkles, too.

In one study, people with very thin, bruise-prone skin were shown to have thicker skin and less bruising after applying Retin-A every night for 3 months. If it works that well, why isn't Retin-A as popular as you might expect? Its biggest drawback is that it can be very irritating if applied right after washing the face. This is why the package directions suggest waiting

20 minutes between cleansing and applying Retin-A. Even so, redness and peeling almost always develop in sensitive areas, especially around the eyes.

In my years of dermatology practice, a number of my patients have reported other disadvantages to using Retin-A. For example:

1. They fell asleep while waiting for the 20 minutes to pass.
2. They kissed somebody with a stubbly beard after applying Retin-A and got a rope-burn-like rash.
3. In some sensitive-skinned patients who applied Retin-A at bedtime, the cream got onto their pillowcases and then around their eyes, causing extensive irritation of the under-eye skin.

Because of complaints such as these, the clever manufacturer of Retin-A developed other retinoid products that aren't so irritating. One milder form, Renova, contains mineral oil in its base. Renova has received FDA approval to be marketed as an antiwrinkle treatment, since the manufacturer did extensive testing to prove its effectiveness in reducing wrinkles. Another retinoid product, Retin-A Micro, has a microsponge delivery system that should minimize irritation by allowing for the time-released absorption of tretinoin.

Though there does appear to be less burning and irritation associated with newer retinoid products, they are about equal in causing *photosensitization*—that is, increasing your sensitivity to the sun. Even if you apply either product at bedtime, your skin will remain very sensitive the next day, making a good zinc-based sunscreen even more necessary.

Another popular prescription retinoid is Tri-Luma, a cream that combines tretinoin with 4 percent hydroquinone. As you'll recall from our discussion of hydroquinone, it's a very effective bleaching ingredient for age spots, brown dots, and masklike stains from pregnancy or oral contraceptives.

Then there is Tazorac, a prescription retinoid that has been promoted primarily as an acne treatment. More recently it's been gaining fame for its antiaging benefits, which is why many dermatologists recommend it to patients. Tazorac is available as a cream or gel that is applied nightly, much like Retin-A—but it seems to be better tolerated.

One nonprescription retinoid, called retinol, can be found in a slew of drugstore and department-store skin-care products. In fact, it has become one of the most popular ingredients in skin rejuvenators. Neutrogena offers an antiwrinkle cream with retinol in its Healthy Skin line, and RoC sells a product called Retinol Correxion; neither one discloses the percentage of retinol. But since retinol is not acidic, it is much better tolerated than Retin-A, Renova, or Tazorac. In my clinical experience, it is also less photosensitizing.

In a study performed by Albert Kligman, MD, the University of Pennsylvania research professor who invented Retin-A, regular nightly use of 0.15 percent retinol reduced the appearance of wrinkles by 30 percent after 1 month. Some physician-strength skin-care products contain retinol in percentages similar to those in the study.

Salicylic Acid

A beta hydroxy acid, or BHA, salicylic acid first appeared in skin-care products—specifically, acne treatments—because it is so good at cleaning out pores. It also happens to be a very effective exfoliant. I like to wash my face with a salicylic acid cleanser because it leaves my skin so clean and refreshed.

In general, salicylic acid is less irritating and better tolerated than glycolic acid. On the other hand, it isn't as effective for reducing facial lines and grooves.

The Olay Age Defying line features several good products that are salicylic based. So is Clinique's best-selling Total Turnaround Cream, which so many of my patients love.

Titanium Dioxide

I truly believe that the cornerstone of great skin care is a titanium dioxide or zinc oxide sunscreen. We can categorize all sun-protection ingredients as either chemical or physical. Simply put, the chemical agents absorb ultraviolet rays, whereas the physical agents deflect UV rays from the skin's surface. The only two physical sun-protection ingredients are titanium dioxide and zinc oxide.

I prefer using the physical agents for their gentleness on the skin, as well as for their ability to block more of the long-wavelength UV rays than the chemical sunscreen agents do. It's important to note that although many skin-care products contain titanium, it provides sun protection only if it's present in an amount significant enough to earn an SPF number.

Vitamin C/Ascorbic Acid

Oral-form vitamin C has long been touted as an effective antioxidant. The topical form became popular after researchers in the Duke University department of dermatology concluded that up to 20 times more vitamin C is absorbed when it concentrates in the skin rather than being taken by mouth.

What does vitamin C do for the skin? In the 1990s, when the topical form became available, it was said to significantly improve the appearance of facial grooves when used for several months. It also seems to have a *photo-protective* effect—that is, it helps protect the skin from the acute damage of sun exposure.

Do I think it works? After examining at least 1,000 patients who have tried various vitamin C formulations, I would say that the topical form by itself does not quickly reduce wrinkles. However, a recent study seems to confirm that topical vitamin C can enhance the effectiveness of sunscreen when people combine the two.

My advice: Try topical vitamin C if you are happy with the improvement from your current skin-care regimen and you want a boost. If you spend a lot of time outdoors, consider applying a vitamin C product under your sunscreen every morning.

Vitamin C oxidizes very rapidly, causing it to turn brown—much like an apple slice left in the open air. We don't know if oxidized vitamin C is as effective as "fresh" vitamin C. To be safe, I suggest storing any vitamin C product in a cool, dark setting—like a medicine cabinet—and away from a hot radiator or an extremely cold window in winter. Also, since vitamin C has a shorter shelf life than other skin-care products, buy it in small quantities or share.

Vitamin K

Some Beauty Campers may have firsthand experience with blood thinners, or *anticoagulants*. These prescription drugs tend to increase the risk of bruising. Vitamin K does the opposite—it helps blood to clot, or coagulate. Applied to the skin, it can prevent bruising and reduce the appearance of dark under-eye circles.

If you're prone to these dark purple circles, broken capillaries on the sides of your nose, or the flush of rosacea, you may want to try a topical vitamin K product. It is also excellent for use before a cosmetic procedure that may result in bruising, like surgery or even injections. If you do end up with bruising from a series of injections, ask your doctor whether topical vitamin K might help clear your skin more quickly.

*Zinc Oxide

The idea of using zinc oxide for sun protection has been around for a long time. Beauty Campers who are baby boomers might remember going to the beach and seeing a lifeguard's lips or nose coated with this gooey white stuff. Zinc oxide also is a long-standing remedy for red or irritated skin. If you've treated a baby for diaper rash, you probably used zinc oxide. It's the active ingredient in almost all diaper rash ointments.

We tend to think of zinc oxide products as heavy and somewhat sticky. The good news is that during the last decade, both zinc oxide and titanium dioxide (another sun-protection ingredient) have become available in more cosmetically acceptable forms. The zinc and titanium now used in skin-care products are nearly invisible, so they don't leave behind a pasty white film when applied to the skin.

Poison Ivy Alert!

Just as I have my favorite skin-care ingredients, I have some not-so-favorites. Typically, these can't do terrible harm; otherwise, we wouldn't see them in so many products. But because all Beauty Campers should know what they're putting on their faces, you will need to learn which ingredients are potentially troublesome and why. Usually it's because they're irritating or comedogenic. (Yes, it's true—some ingredients can cause acne!) So, Beauty Campers, if you ever develop a mystery rash or a sudden acne flare-up, you'll be able to identify the potential culprits.

One of these questionable ingredients is *lanolin*. This wool derivative, sometimes called wool alcohol, is an effective moisturizer, or humectant. Lanolin can be found in brand-name body lotions such as Eucerin, as well as in cosmetics from Almay and Clinique. Unfortunately, lanolin also is one of the most common irritants in skin-care products. In fact, it's one of the 24 ingredients for which dermatologists routinely do allergy testing.

How can you tell if you may be allergic to lanolin? If, like me, you become very red and itchy when wearing wool, that's your first sign of possible trouble. If you can wear wool without problem but notice some unexplained redness, flakiness, or another possible symptom of a skin rash, you might want to try this at-home version of a dermatologist's patch test. (Many people can wear wool but can't tolerate certain lanolin products.)

Find an area of your body where you can apply the product in question as directed for 5 to 7 days. It should be somewhere that has skin similar to your facial skin, but not your face or neck. Above the crease of the elbow and on the inside of the upper arm (near the crease of the underarm) are good test spots. If you don't notice any adverse reaction in the designated time period, then that particular lanolin product isn't causing the problem. However, it doesn't mean that another product isn't the culprit. Each lanolin product varies in strength and ability to cause irritation. Someone with sensitive skin would be wise to do a patch test with each new product before applying it to her face.

Two more questionable ingredients are *sodium lauryl sulfate* and *ammonium lauryl sulfate*, both of which I suggest avoiding. They're the foaming agents in most bubble baths and nonsoap cleansers, including the priciest products. Often little girls who like to soak in bubble baths end up with inflamed bottoms, the result of a reaction to one of the lauryl sulfates. These ingredients can wreak the same havoc when applied to the face. To add insult to injury, the lauryl sulfates are comedogenic. By all means, steer clear of products containing either of these ingredients.

In response to consumer complaints, many manufacturers have switched from the lauryl sulfates to a similar but harmless foaming agent called sodium laureth sulfate. I know it might seem a bit confusing, but believe me, that *eth* ending can make all the difference in the world. Products with sodium laur*eth* sulfate seldom aggravate the skin.

Then there's the ever-popular *shea butter*, a moisturizing agent found in loads of skin-care products and advertised as something truly sensational and "natural." Once I had the unfortunate experience of using a hair mask that contained shea butter. (I didn't read the ingredient label, if you can imagine that!) As all hair-care products do, this one eventually traveled to my face—probably via my pillowcase or hands. Shea butter can be a major pore-clogger. In my case, I broke out with painful, almost cystic acne.

Ironically, *benzoyl peroxide*—one of the tried-and-true acne remedies—can cause problems for its devotees. Before the advent of the Proactiv antiacne line, many dermatologists would instruct patients to be cautious about using benzoyl peroxide, because it left a lot of people with dry, red, irritated skin. Then Kathy Fields, MD, and Katie Rodan, MD, tried something new. They made benzoyl peroxide in a lower strength— about half the strength of many of the products available in drugstores at the time. It worked, and it was far less irritating than other benzoyl peroxide products. Not surprisingly, the Proactiv line has become wildly popular.

My only caveat with Proactiv and similar products: Although benzoyl peroxide is a terrific antiacne ingredient, I recommend taking breaks from it. Many of my own patients notice a dramatic reduction in redness once they discontinue the very same benzoyl peroxide product that at one time helped so much.

Last, to those with sensitive skin, a word of caution about using botanicals: I know these ingredients smell nice, but just because they're natural doesn't mean they can't cause problems. An episode of *Grey's Anatomy*—one of my favorite TV shows— perfectly illustrates this point. The "patient," Mrs. McDreamy, had relieved herself in the woods while walking her dog and ended up with a terrible case of blisters on her bottom. It seems that while squatting, she inadvertently rubbed against one mysterious leaf too many!

I often compare skin-care formulations that contain five or more botanicals to a day in the woods: You never know what will happen when you rub the product onto a sensitive area like your face or neck (or even your bottom). With so many potentially troublesome ingredients, you certainly are more likely to experience an unpleasant reaction to one of them!

So read your ingredient labels carefully. When in doubt, patch-test a product for 5 to 7 days in a place where a reaction won't be a problem.

WEEK #2 REVIEW

- *Collect all of your skin-care products and sort them into three piles: Not-Sures, Discards, and Essentials.*
- *Swap and share products with your fellow Beauty Campers.*
- *Know what you should expect from a product—and make sure that it delivers on its claims.*
- *Study the labels of products in your Not-Sure and Essential piles, paying particular attention to the lists of ingredients.*
- *Learn to trust an ingredient, not a brand name.*
- *Familiarize yourself with my favorite ingredients.*
- *Be careful with the "poison ivy" ingredients—and avoid sodium lauryl sulfate and ammonium lauryl sulfate altogether.*
- *Make sure that you're getting 30 minutes more sleep a night. (Your pictures won't lie!)*
- *Keep doing those facial exercises.*

Week #3

Your New Regimen

This week's agenda:
Putting your daily regimen together

Dear Beauty Camper, how well do you know yourself? This is important, because your ability to create a skin-care regimen—and to follow through with it—depends on how accurately you can assess your own needs and preferences. This isn't about ingredients or about your Uninvited Elements (UEs). It is about your mind-set.

You can't transform your skin just by reading this book. Consider it a call to action, with the goal of designing a regimen that's effective, affordable, easily sustainable—even fun! By taking into account your perception and philosophy of skin care, your new regimen will achieve the right balance—not just for your face but for your life.

We'll begin with what's familiar to you: your current skin-care regimen, with the products that you identified in Week #2 as Essentials and Not-Sures. By reading labels, weeding out ineffective or troublesome products, and applying your new knowledge of beneficial ingredients, we will gradually upgrade your regimen to better suit you.

Before we move ahead, I want to remind you of a few changes that you already should have adopted. If you haven't already done so, now is the time to buy that high-quality, 400-thread-count, 100 percent cotton pillowcase that will be gentle to your skin while you sleep. And remember to wash your pillowcase—along with the rest of your bedding and your washcloths and towels—in All Free Clear laundry detergent. You won't believe how much kinder they'll be to your face, especially if you have sensitive or easily irritated skin.

Another important change is to get in the habit of washing your face with cool or tepid water. It won't aggravate your skin or cause redness and broken capillaries, as hot water can.

You may want to invest in a high-wattage lightbulb for your bathroom—as long as it isn't fluorescent, which tends to cast an awful tint on the skin. I laugh when I see my face in the mirror under the harsh fluorescent lighting of my exam rooms. Suffice it to say, I don't look my best.

I also recommend picking up a nice, full shower cap. You'll be surprised by how much better your hair behaves and how much less dry it feels when you protect it from humidity and moisture as you wash your face or take a shower.

For creams and other leave-on treatments that you might use after you've cleansed your face, remember that the order of application doesn't matter. The smallest molecules penetrate and travel to the dermis first, while the larger molecules penetrate more slowly. This is true regardless of when you apply something or whether you slather it on top of five other products. Lipids don't penetrate at all. Their job is to remain on the surface of the skin, protecting it and preventing water from escaping.

Okay. Now that we've recapped what I consider the basics of good skin care, let's turn our attention to you—your personality, your perspective on skin care, and your strength of desire for improvement. All of these will influence your decisions and choices during the rest of Beauty Camp.

CAMP ACTIVITY #1

WHAT KIND OF BEAUTY CAMPER ARE YOU?

Real progress in anything requires self-awareness and candor, not romantic ideals. Before you can make real progress in rebuilding your skin-care regimen, you will need to determine what type of Beauty Camper you are.

The Gung Ho Camper: Some campers could spend hours in front of the bathroom or vanity mirror. They love to shop for new skin-care products, experiment with them, and gab about them with friends. They might make discreet trips to beauty boutiques and hide the shopping bags from their partners. They know the names of all the good spas around the country (whether or not they've been to them) and occasionally fantasize about designing their own line of toiletry bags because they can't seem to find one that's big enough.

My hunch is that a good number of women who buy this book fall into this category. They constantly are on the prowl for new approaches to looking better. But here's the hitch: A Gung Ho Camper might have trouble sticking with a skin-care regimen because she is always tempted to run off and try another. She's a sampler, a tester, a gadfly in the cosmetic aisle.

Does this sound anything like you? If so, please make an extra effort to commit to the skin-care regimen that you are about to start. Think of yourself as being on a journey—but you need to stay in one place long enough to find out what it's really like.

The Too-Busy Camper: For this camper, tending to her appearance is a responsibility or an obligation—not something that she enjoys. She probably doesn't have lots of free time; perhaps she juggles a family and a full-time job. She might be more worried about her weight than her face and would rather spend a spare half hour swimming, bicycling, or practicing yoga. Isn't that more important, anyway?

This camper may be a bit on the skeptical side. She can rarely squeeze in a workout at the gym, and now she's supposed to do exercises for her face? Never mind the ridiculous notion that she can get 30 more minutes of sleep each night.

Here's the funny thing: The Too-Busy Camper is just the sort who really will stick with her skin-care regimen once she has made a commitment to it. Give her a task, and she'll follow through. It's almost as though her worries about not having enough time magically create more.

The Bad-Attitude Camper: At one time this camper may have spent lots of time on her appearance, experimenting with makeup or hairstyles. But somewhere along the way, she lost interest. Now she could care less about looking better (except when a stranger asks if her husband is her son!). She dreads the prospect of leaning over the sink and splashing off one more acid product in the hope of seeing some improvement in her skin. Her new mantra is "Appearance isn't everything." In her view, in fact, it isn't anything at all.

This camper probably came to Beauty Camp at the behest of her mother, sister, or friend. She'd rather not be here because she's "too busy" to bother with any of it. But her ambivalence about her appearance may be a subconscious way of protecting herself from possibly disappointing results. If she can't look perfect, she reasons, why try at all?

If this sounds like you, I have a counterintuitive suggestion: Start with a few more products and a slightly more complex skin-care regimen than the Gung Ho Camper who loves to experiment. But skip the Extreme Challenges that you'll encounter later in this book. They definitely aren't for you.

So . . . which Beauty Camper best describes you? I don't mean to suggest that every woman easily fits into one category or another. My point is this: Even if simple strategies like buying new pillowcases and getting more sleep can lead to dramatic improvement in your appearance, they won't work for you if they don't suit your fundamental personality. And your personality isn't going to change. So accept yourself, embrace yourself—even laugh at yourself—and try to devise a daily skin-care regimen that won't have you struggling against your own nature.

Games Campers Play

There's an ideal combination of products for your skin, your attitude, and your budget. Finding that combination is easy. Sticking with it can be more difficult, depending on your personality. But with a few clever tools and techniques, you can motivate and even outsmart yourself to stay on track.

Over the years, I've resorted to my own bag of tricks for just this purpose. On one occasion, after an extended visit to Italy with my family, I stepped onto a pharmacy scale, only to discover that I had gained 8 pounds while traveling. Did I notice my thickening waist? Not really. I thought I looked terrific—particularly in the photos from our trip, which had been shot from the waist up. (My husband, Rob, kept telling me that I was looking more like Sophia Loren every day!)

When I arrived home, very well rested, my older female patients also told me that I looked wonderful. I explained that I'd gained weight by eating my way through Italy. They unanimously concluded that the extra pounds made my face look great. Encouraged by this, I didn't bother to diet. In fact, I just kept eating.

It wasn't long before the extra pounds took a toll on my weak back. And even though my face appeared to have fewer lines, I realized that from the waist down, I looked pretty awful. *No problem*, I told myself. *I can lose the weight in no time. After all, I needed just a little over a month to gain it.* So I tried and tried, for almost a year. Nothing worked. I just couldn't get motivated.

Adopting a new tack, I recruited my husband to diet with me, since he'd gained a hefty sum, too. We started by taking pictures of ourselves. That seemed like a good idea. We even put on bathing suits. My husband took a couple of random Polaroids of me, full body, in an old bikini left over from my prepregnancy days.

Honestly, at the moment the camera's flash went off, I didn't have any game plan to lose weight. I just knew instinctively that if I saw an unedited, unforgiving photo of myself, I might be motivated to accomplish what I hadn't succeeded in doing for almost a year. And you know, it worked!

Rob and I posted our photos in our bathroom. I lost the extra pounds in a couple of months just by counting calories.

The truth is, faced with the reality of that photo every morning and night, I had little problem eating smaller amounts, often leaving some food on my plate (since I do think that American portions are too large in the first place).

No diet—and I had tried them all—did for me what those photos did. Six years later, they remain in a place of honor above our medicine cabinet mirror. The experience left me with an even greater appreciation of this wonderful expression: Nothing tastes as good as looking fit feels.

Are you gung ho at the start of projects but unable to stick with them? Do you lose interest easily? Or are you just too busy to pay attention to your skin-care regimen? You might try taping a particularly craggy Orientation photo in your bathroom, where you can't avoid seeing it every day. You also might start out with a very basic, bare-bones regimen of no more than three products, adding a new one every other week or so. That should help keep you motivated. And the Extreme Challenges along the way definitely are for you.

My Own Daily Regimen

You also are more likely to stick with your skin-care regimen if it's engaging to you. How you define "engaging" is up to you. It may mean streamlining your current regimen—or adding more products. It's a reality: What may seem like too many products and too complex a daily or weekly regimen for one person might be simple and straightforward to another. For example, I have no problem at all using 11 or 12 products every day. That's right: a full dozen!

My at-home regimen might seem ridiculous and overly complicated to some. But after years of experimentation—there isn't a skin-care product or procedure that I recommend to a patient that I haven't tried myself—I feel that I've created a program that really works for me. Here's what it entails.

1. In the morning, I get out of bed and take a shower in warm, but not too hot, water. I wash my face with a gentle nonsoap cleanser that contains salicylic acid. I never use soap because of the redness and scaling that it can cause. (My cleanser is the product that I rotate most, as you will see when we discuss Survival Basics in just a bit.) I get out of the shower and pat my skin dry.

2. I apply a film of a nondrying gel mask with an oxygen activator to my face—including a smudge under my eyebrows—as well as under my chin and on my neck and chest. After breakfast, I organize myself for the day, choosing my clothes and such. Within 20 to 30 minutes, I rinse off the gel.

3. I spread a single drop of neuropeptide onto my forehead, another around my eyes and lips, and a third into my frown lines and neck. Then I apply a thin film of lipids all over, along with an antipuff peptide serum just under my eyes. That's followed by an algae peptide cream with antioxidants and glycolic acid, which goes over my entire face. To my neck and chest, I apply a cream with lipids, lactic acid, peptides, and an antioxidant all in one. Finally, I put a zinc-based SPF 36 sunscreen all over my face, my neck, and any parts of my chest that will be exposed to the sun that day. The sunscreen contains Colhibin and Elhibin, which help diminish the appearance of lines.

4. I wait a minute for everything to soak in, sometimes while I'm getting dressed. Then I do my eye makeup and lipstick, applying another light coating of algae peptide cream on my lips for good measure. A dab of mineral powder on my nose, and I'm ready to go. I don't use any foundation or face makeup; with the health and quality of my skin, I really have no need for it. After all the time I've spent making sure that my pores are clear, my skin tone is even, and the surface is clean, why should I hide it?

In the evening, my regimen changes a little. Before going to bed, I use a makeup remover with hyaluronic acid, which conditions my eyelashes, brows, and lids. Sometimes I apply a papaya scrub for exfoliating and softening my skin. On other nights—particularly in the summer when I've had a superlong day—I might go for some kind of cooling, tightening mask with camphor, cucumber, or menthol.

The funny thing is, at one time I didn't believe in masks. But I've grown to love them as I've gotten older. And my kids discovered the benefits of masks much sooner than I did. When my youngest daughter, Liza, invites friends over, they like to apply a pumpkin mask that I've formulated. This particular one gives great "instant gratification" in terms of cleaning out pores.

At bedtime, after I rinse and pat dry my face, I repeat my morning regimen, without the sunscreen. I add a fade lotion that contains algae peptides, hydroquinone, and glycolic acid. It evens my skin tone, promotes collagen and elastin production, reduces fine lines, and plumps up the surface of my skin. On top of everything, I might put lipids and my oxygen-activating mask, which is light enough for me to sleep in.

For an extra nighttime boost, I apply 0.3 percent retinol two or three times a week, as my skin can tolerate it. I use it as a spot treatment, really—and never every night. Retinol isn't considered a new ingredient anymore, but it has proven highly effective, and I think most women will want to try it at some point. You can start with a drugstore or department-store brand, most of which are about 0.005 percent retinol. A "physician-strength" formula, like the one I use, can be 10 to 20 times stronger.

I'm not going to lie to you: Mine is a take-no-prisoners approach. But my appearance is vital to my career and livelihood. As I've learned over the years, it truly affects how others respond to me and how I feel about myself.

That said, you shouldn't rush out to duplicate my regimen. While it works for me, it may not be right for you. Besides, you don't want to buy jars and bottles harum-scarum, only to find yourself overwhelmed by a confusing array of stuff—and no idea of what do with it. Instead, think simple to start.

It's a little like learning how to cook. The first time you try to make a new dish, you find an easy recipe and follow the directions. As you grow more confident and adept, you can experiment and improvise.

CAMP ACTIVITY #2
YOUR WISH LIST

Once you've studied your Orientation photos (in Week #1) and my list of favorite ingredients (Week #2), you're ready to come up with your own wish list for rejuvenating your face and fighting your UEs. This list can be as long as you want—just like the one you'd give to Santa Claus (and just as expensive).

You might go on an exploratory mission, taking an afternoon to survey the skin-care products currently on the market. You could do this with other Beauty Campers, if you like, organizing a field trip to a cosmetics warehouse or large beauty boutique. This really will help you put together your wish list.

Hit the drugstore, the "personal care" aisle at the supermarket, and all the department stores in the mall (they don't carry the same product lines). Open those tester bottles and jars! Smell everything! Try everything! Ask for free samples and trial sizes. Interview some of the sales staff and ask for their personal recommendations. Everybody has at least one product they swear by.

If you know a good aesthetician or a skin-care specialist in a dermatologist's office or at a day spa, you might ask this person to accompany you on your excursion. Perhaps you have a friend who stays up-to-date on skin-care ingredients and formulations. Pick her brain, too.

Take a notepad and pencil when you're interviewing skin-care professionals or knowledgeable laywomen. Write down the names of their recommended products, as well as the ingredients. Also note the prices of these products from store to store. They can really vary.

Do not buy anything on this trip. We aren't quite ready.

Setting a Reasonable Budget—and Program

After your exploratory mission, you should have a good sense of what skin-care products cost. And you probably realize that you could spend anywhere from $40 a month to $400. I know these numbers may sound scary, but think back to Week #2 of Beauty Camp, when you added up the prices of all those products in your box. How much are you spending already?

Now comes the moment of truth: You need to reach an agreement with yourself about how much you're willing and able to spend. Please don't overextend yourself. Remember: There's a regimen for every budget—and sometimes the cheapest ones work the best.

It's almost time to create your shopping list. But first, a reminder: The last thing you should do is try to duplicate my regimen—or anybody else's, for that matter. Your skin care is too important to be dictated by another person. This is why you must do some basic research and make your own decisions. Never, ever buy anything solely on blind faith, a marketing campaign—or even my opinion.

If you are feeling unsure and want to move ahead more cautiously or are worried about blowing your budget, I strongly urge you to find friends who'll chip in for certain products and share, say, an expensive jar of peptide cream or a high-strength glycolic acid gel. Again, it's smart to ask for small trial sizes of new products. The salespeople at department-store cosmetics counters tend to be pretty generous with their samples. Sometimes they'll give you a few of them at once, enough to last a week or two—just a fair amount of time to see if a product does what it should.

If you're a Gung Ho Camper, you need to be extra-careful not to overdo it. Start even simpler than you may be inclined to. This will allow you to judge which products are working and which aren't. If you try too many new things at once, you may not be able to distinguish among their effects. Also, some Beauty Campers who go overboard and buy lots of products quickly lose interest and don't stick with their regimens long enough to see results. This is a waste of time and money—and the reason that so many people lose faith in either a product or the skin-care professional who recommended it. Pretty soon, they've moved on to another miracle cure.

Finding the Right Ingredients for You

Remember, the promise of a product is driven by the ingredients, not by the package. Don't fall for sexy boxes, bottles, and jars. The label tells the whole story.

Which products you choose for your basic skin-care regimen will depend on your goals. In broad brushstrokes:

- If you want to minimize pores, use glycolic and salicylic acids.
- If you want to reduce dynamic lines, use a neuropeptide.
- If you want to revive dull skin, use a microdermabrasion or exfoliating product.
- If you want firmer skin, use a peptide and gradually introduce a retinoid—even if only for twice-a-week applications.
- If you want to counteract environmental damage (from sun exposure, smoking, stress, or excessive alcohol consumption, among other lifestyle factors), use an antioxidant product.

As we discussed in Week #2, pay especially close attention to the sequence of ingredients on the label. On most products, ingredients appear in descending order by amount or concentration. This probably is as close as you'll get to discerning how much of an ingredient is present, since most products don't specify percentages.

For example, if you're shopping for a glycolic acid product, you'll want a formulation with enough glycol (at least 5 percent) to make a noticeable difference in your skin. If glycolic acid appears last in the ingredient list or even in the third-to-last place, you are probably getting less than 1 percent glycolic acid. You may want to consider a physician-strength formula, which you can order by phone or online and shouldn't require an office visit.

If you tend to have large pores or breakouts, be sure to avoid any skin-care products with shea butter, lanolin, or sodium lauryl sulfate.

Equipped with this information, some Beauty Campers may be ready to go shopping for skin-care products. Others may want more detailed guidelines on putting together a simple but effective regimen. If this describes you, then proceed to the "Survival Basics" below. These basics will empower you to move ahead with confidence—and keep you from going broke.

Survival Basics

At a bare minimum, there are five fundamentals to an effective skin-care regimen: cleansing, exfoliating, moisturizing, rejuvenating (the meaning of which will vary, depending on your skin's current condition), and protecting. I call these the Survival Basics. All of them can be accomplished with just one or two products—or a whole basketful. Your budget and the degree of complexity with which you're comfortable will steer you toward your own skin-care regimen.

With this in mind, here are some guidelines for choosing products in each of the Survival Basic categories.

1. CLEANSING

First, please discard any bar soap that you may be using now. Soaps are alkaline products that work by removing the skin's oil and lipids. Washing your face with soap can result in dryness, redness, and irritation.

Instead, look for a simple, nonsoap liquid cleanser (made from water, glycerin, and a foaming agent) or a cleansing cream (a nonfoaming product made from water, botanical or mineral oils, petrolatum, and waxes). Both products leave lipids on the skin's surface and, therefore, are less likely to cause dryness, redness, or irritation. The nonsoap liquids are better at cleansing the skin's surface, but they aren't very moisturizing. The creams are moisturizing but generally less antibacterial. For this reason, I usually don't recommend cleansing creams for people with acne or inflamed rosacea.

Changes in season—or changes in your lifestyle or activity level—may require a change in cleansers. In the summer, for example, you might want to try a salicylic acid cleanser, which can get into your pores and really clear them of debris. A winter cold snap or ski trip might warrant a shift to a gentler, more moisturizing cleanser. If you have trouble with acne in the winter, I'd switch to a benzoyl peroxide cleanser for its antiacne and antibacterial properties, then follow up with a botanical cleanser if your skin feels dry. This routine works well for many of my female patients; it's much like shampooing and then conditioning your hair.

I prefer washing my face with my clean hands. If you want to increase the exfoliation of dead skin cells, you can use a disposable Buf-Puf or a washcloth. Please remember to wash the cloth in your washer's hot cycle at least once a week. This will prevent bacterial overgrowth on the surface.

Also, when you wash your face, please be sure to go all the way to your hairline. This is important to remove all of the residue from your hair-care products.

If cleansing seems a bit complex, rest assured, it really isn't. Here's a quick summary of the key points.

- Always use a nonsoap cleanser without lauryl sulfate.
- When your skin is dry, consider using a cleansing cream, which is moisturizing.
- When your skin is oily, switch to a salicylic acid cleanser. This is also your best choice if you're in a hot or humid climate, where you tend to perspire more.
- If you have active acne, use benzoyl peroxide (for a limited period of time), glycolic acid, or salicylic acid for cleansing.
- If your skin is suffering a bit from a certain physical activity, like swimming, consider using a moisturizing botanical cleanser.
- If you wear a lot of makeup, be sure that your nighttime cleanser adequately removes all makeup residue. If it doesn't, you may want to use a separate makeup remover,

so your skin is able to absorb all those great skin-care products while you sleep. My favorite makeup removers contain their own good ingredients, like hyaluronic acid, so I can "condition" my lashes and eyebrows as I remove my mascara and brow powder.

* Rotate your cleansers as needed, depending on seasonal changes, your skin's condition due to lifestyle or activity level, and stress or hormonal fluctuations.

2. EXFOLIATING

When you were young, your mother might have instructed you to scrub your face. You probably thought (as I did) that you were getting rid of dirt. In fact, you were also clearing away dead cells from the skin's surface. That's the idea behind exfoliation: the removal of clumps of dead cells, along with the debris, oil, and excess pigment that cling to these cells.

If you're fortunate enough to not have acne, enlarged pores, uneven pigment, or generally lackluster skin, then you may not need to exfoliate at this time. In my experience, however, it's a rare person who isn't at least somewhat bothered by one or more of these problems at certain times of the month or during certain seasons of the year.

When dead cells accumulate on the surface, the skin looks duller, rougher, drier, and flakier. Some cells may clog pores, causing the pores to stretch out—making them larger and eventually producing whiteheads and blackheads. Good exfoliation will brighten and smooth the skin's surface, improving a lackluster appearance, shrinking pores, and preventing breakouts. It can also help clear acne and inflamed rosacea lesions.

Another important reason to exfoliate: The dead cells act as a coat of armor on your skin, preventing your new products from penetrating to a layer where they can do the most good.

Skin-care products exfoliate in one of two ways: chemically, with salicylic or glycolic acid (among other alpha hydroxy acids) or a retinoid; or physically, using particles that are abrasive or that bead on your face. Just as there are chemical exfoliants of varying strengths (due to different acid concentrations), there are physical exfoliants of varying strengths. If you study the labels of microdermabrasion creams and scrubs, you will notice that the exfoliating ingredients range from very abrasive (like apricot or walnut kernels or cornmeal, which can irritate sensitive skin) to gentle (tiny balls or beads, the most popular being jojoba beads).

You probably have some experience with scrubs. Do you like the way they feel? While you are out on your exploratory mission to check out skin-care products, you might want to look for various exfoliants and ask for samples. Squeeze the abrasive types onto your hand so you can feel how rough they are.

In addition to acidic cleansers and microdermabrasion creams and scrubs, you can exfoliate with a leave-on product, such as a day cream with a good exfoliating ingredient: glycolic acid, salicylic acid, or a retinoid.

If you're feeling timid or your skin tends to be sensitive and acne prone, tread carefully into the world of exfoliants. I would start by using a beaded scrub or a wash-off glycolic acid product. Then, as your skin acclimates to the glycolic acid, you can add a gentle leave-on product for nighttime.

Some Beauty Campers will prefer the simplicity of an exfoliating cleanser, while others might seek the extra benefits of a leave-on agent, like a glycolic acid toner or gel. Remember, too, that anything capable of scrubbing your face is a potential exfoliating implement. Washcloths, sponges, and Buf-Pufs are good for exfoliating and easy to come by. There also are brand-

Too Much of a Strong Thing!

I didn't get serious about exfoliating until I was on the brink of 40. Now it's part of my daily routine. And I truly believe that my skin looks better at 53 than it did at 39!

Because my skin is very sensitive, I do need to carefully tread the line between good exfoliation and overworking my skin. You might need to be mindful of this, too. Remember: If you develop any redness or irritation, or if you feel even the least bit sensitive in any area, do not apply an exfoliating product to that area until your symptoms improve. Then, when you resume exfoliating, do it less often—perhaps at one-third the frequency.

Let's say that while you're using an exfoliating cream, the skin beneath your eyes becomes red and irritated. Stop applying your cream in that area until your skin clears. Then you can resume using the cream—but only in sparing amounts and only every third night for a week. If your skin seems to tolerate this, step up to every other night— and be sure to keep monitoring for an adverse reaction. Plenty of exfoliants are quite effective when used just several times a week.

name microdermabrasion kits marketed with the promise that they fight acne and wrinkles all at once.

Whatever your exfoliant of choice, please take care not to get overzealous with it. A big raw patch on your face is far more unsightly—not to mention painful—than a few lines.

3. MOISTURIZING

Until the 1970s, moisturizing was the main thrust of the leave-on products in skin-care regimens. These products grew out of the traditional notion of cold creams. But an old-fashioned cold cream, which is a petroleum- and water-based product, functions like a hand cream. It can protect against raw, flaky skin—surface dryness—but it cannot prevent or diminish lines.

These days, what you're looking for in a moisturizer is much more than just a cream. Some daytime moisturizing formulas contain sunscreen. Others contain antiaging ingredients. For starters, you want something that—if nothing else—is proven to hydrate the skin. By "hydrate," I mean that the product helps hold water in your skin, keeping it plump and fresh looking.

Just how do moisturizers increase the water content of skin cells? As you might guess, the answer lies in the ingredients.

Blocking Water Loss with Lipids

Lipids are the perennial best-selling ingredient in the skin-care line I've formulated for physicians to sell—beating out dozens of other worthy products. Why? These oils are natural to our skin.

When we're born, lipids create a barrier film (much like plastic wrap) on the skin's surface to trap water. This in part is why a baby's face is so smooth and soft. But from childhood on, lipid levels diminish, resulting in a loss of smoothness and softness.

Many people turn to lipids as their skin becomes drier, which they often perceive as one of the first signs of aging. But even my son Danny, who is in his early twenties, swears by the lipids that he applies twice a day to his face.

Interestingly, cholesterol-lowering drugs seem to affect lipid levels in the skin, causing it to become very dry over time. If you are taking one of these medications, you may want to consider moisturizing with topical lipids. Likewise, people with dry-skin conditions, like childhood eczema, do very well by using lipid-containing products.

Among the lipids naturally found in the skin are ceramides, cholesterol, and sphingolipids. The good news is that lipids made in the laboratory can be incorporated into your skin-care regimen. When used every day, they keep skin looking healthy and vibrant. The grandma of all lipid products, Elizabeth Arden's Ceramide, is still going strong. A great new drugstore line called CeraVe—which includes a cleanser, lotion, and cream—features multiple ceramides and cholesterol. And it's very reasonably priced.

Plumping with Humectants

Other popular ingredients that you might look for in moisturizing products go by the scientific name *humectants*. These attract water from the environment and produce a net increase in water content at the skin's surface, creating the appearance of smoother skin.

A very good and popular humectant is hyaluronic acid. As I mentioned in Week #2, this ingredient is very much like a sponge, able to hold 1,000 times its weight in water. For this reason, it makes a very good surface moisturizer. Its molecules are too large to penetrate to the dermis, so it can't replace the hyaluronic acid that we produce naturally but lose to sun damage. (In the Beauty Camp Extra on page 207, we'll discuss Restylane, an injectable form of hyaluronic acid that doctors can administer directly into deeper facial grooves to instantly fill and lift them.)

Another common humectant is collagen, which—like hyaluronic acid—has large molecules that can't reach the dermal skin layer. Since it can hold only 20 times its weight in water—much less than hyaluronic acid—it really isn't the preferable humectant ingredient, in my opinion. (Similarly, injectable collagen lasts a shorter time and produces less dramatic results then Restylane.)

Going Deep

Some ingredients in skin-care formulas consist of molecules that are small enough to penetrate to the living skin cells of the epidermis. This isn't snake oil; it's real science. In fact, very small, lightweight molecules can travel as deep as the interface between the epidermis and the dermis, the so-called epidemal-dermal junction. Other ingredients produce changes deep in the skin by sending messenger molecules into the dermis to stimulate the manufacture of key skin components.

Studies have shown that both glycolic acid and retinoids increase the production of hyaluronic acid in the dermis. Algae peptides also are able to affect this deepest skin layer. In clinical trials, twice-daily application of 5 percent algae peptides improved hydration of the skin by 128 percent after just 4 weeks. But now we've wandered into our next Survival Basic: rejuvenating.

4. REJUVENATING

In the trendy world of skin care, marketers seem to be abandoning the term *rejuvenating* in favor of *antiaging*. This is because consumers should put their efforts into preventing skin aging, rather than waiting until they need to undo age-related changes.

Still, I prefer *rejuvenation*. For one thing, why should we "antiage"? This seems silly to me. I'm proud of my age because so much richness has come with the years.

Besides, aging is inevitable, whether or not I have lines on my face. The only thing that can truly stop the aging process is death. Am I right? So for me, the word of choice is *rejuvenation*. Believe it or not, but some of the newer skin-care products really can rejuvenate tired, sagging skin. With so many ingredients proven to rid skin cells of damaging free radicals, reduce the depth of wrinkles, and even restore collagen, who wouldn't want to take advantage of them?

If the world of exfoliants seemed a little complex initially, prepare yourself for the galaxy of rejuvenating skin-care products currently on the market. Just stay with me; I promise that choosing the best product for you will become simpler.

As with cleansing and exfoliating, you have a number of effective options for rejuvenating skin. Which one you choose for your basic regimen should depend on your primary concerns about your skin. Here are some general guidelines.

The Truth about Skin Type

I am 100 percent Italian, an ethnicity known for its ability to tan beautifully. Yet I'm very fair skinned. Until I was in my twenties, I could hardly be out in the sun without getting a very bad burn. On my first trip to Florida, I decided to go sunbathing at 5 o'clock in the afternoon, when the sun's rays no longer are at their strongest. I stayed out for an hour—and ended up with blisters up and down my legs!

Most well-trained dermatologists will tell you that someone who always burns and never tans cannot get brown discoloration on her skin. Guess what? I always have, even since my early childhood. This tendency toward staining undoubtedly is rooted in my Italian heritage. The point I want to make to you is that no one—no one—can know your skin better than you do, once you educate yourself and hone your observational skills.

The concept of "skin type," such as a dermatologist might use it ("always burns, never tans" or "always tans, never burns"), is formally known as the Fitzpatrick skin-typing system. It's named for its creator, Thomas Fitzpatrick, MD, PhD, who was chairman of the department of dermatology at Harvard Medical School during my brother Michael's residency there. "Fitz" himself had five kids, and he was very fatherly toward my brother.

After my first year of medical school, I went to work at Harvard under the supervision of John Parrish, MD, who is the present chair of the department of dermatology.

Although I spent most of my time in Dr. Parrish's lab, my brother supervised a skin surgery clinic once a week, which he invited me to come and observe. I was all of 22 at the time; I still thought of my brother as Mikey, not Dr. Michael Caruso.

One morning, as I stood in the hallway of this bustling and very austere institution, I spotted my brother in the hall. I yelled, "Hey, Mikey, can you come on over here?" That got the attention of Dr. Fitzpatrick, who approached me with very raised eyebrows.

"What is your name, Dr. Caruso's sister?"

"Loretta Caruso," I said. "Sorry if I was a bit loud."

"Loretta Caruso," he replied. "You're wearing that white coat for a reason. So let's give you a project to do." He found a blank piece of paper. "I want you to professionally interview every single patient who walks in the door. You are going to ask them about their skin. Let's see—if they always burn, never tan, let's call that skin type I. . . ."

That was the birth of the Fitzpatrick skin-typing system and my small role in it. True, Fitzpatrick typing can help us doctors keep certain patients out of harm's way—for example, by not using lasers on those who are Fitzpatrick type IV and above. But what I've learned from interviewing my own patients in the more than 3 ensuing decades is this: Only we ourselves can understand what skin type we have—and none of us fits neatly into a doctor-created cubbyhole!

To reduce the appearance of fine lines and deeper wrinkles: You may want to look for a product that contains peptides. Some peptides can produce firmer-looking skin after just one use. Another nonprescription ingredient that helps to diminish lines and deeper wrinkles is retinol. In a study by Albert Kligman, MD, the father of Retin-A, using 0.15 percent retinol decreased the appearance of wrinkles by about 30 percent.

To improve dynamic lines: You can't beat a good neuropeptide for what are sometimes called *personality lines*, like crow's-feet or the frown line between your eyebrows. A neuropeptide is also terrific for filling out lip lines. In fact, continued use can provide a better overall lip appearance. One caveat: You should apply a neuropeptide only in the areas where you want to diminish lines—not all over your face.

To combat tired skin: Smokers, insomniacs, and people under a lot of stress are especially vulnerable to damaging free radicals. For them, an antioxidant product is the best choice for restoring healthy, vibrant skin.

To fade age spots: We'll cover this more completely in Week #4. For now, if you have age spots or other skin discolorations because of a past pregnancy or oral contraceptive use, you'll want to try a product that contains hydroquinone, the best fade ingredient. (Please note that you should not use hydroquinone during preganancy.)

The good news: Most skin-care products offer a combination of rejuvenating ingredients. Depending on your primary skin concerns, it might be wise to start with a product that covers a lot of ground—such as an alpha hydroxy acid with peptides, retinol, antioxidants, and even hydroquinone.

5. PROTECTING

The fifth and final Survival Basic is a zinc-based sunscreen. You'd be smart to find a daytime moisturizer that's both rejuvenating and sun protecting. It will prevent sun damage and, therefore, age spots and freckles. As a bonus, the zinc oxide will calm your skin and reduce any redness brought on by the hormonal fluctuations associated with oral contraceptives, perimenopause, and certainly menopause. (Actually, women who take hormone replacement therapy to manage menopausal symptoms often find that the estrogens cause blotching of their skin.)

When people ask which sunscreen I recommend, I tell them to find one that they really like—the scent, the thickness, the texture, its appearance on the skin. If a sunscreen stings your eyes or has an unpleasant smell, you'll never use it!

In general, tinted sunscreens are the most popular among my patients, since these products give the skin a good "finish" in addition to protecting and moisturizing. If you are using a zinc-based sunscreen, you probably will prefer one with a tint, because it won't leave behind the familiar white cast that even the "clear" Z-Cote (zinc oxide) products can cause.

CAMP ACTIVITY #3
MAKING YOUR SHOPPING LIST

Using the Survival Basics as your guide, you're ready to assemble your shopping list for skin-care products. I would encourage you to carry this book with you when you go shopping. If that isn't convenient for you, at least make a photocopy of the following list.

- Cleanse: _____
- Exfoliate: _____
- Moisturize: _____
- Rejuvenate: _____
- Protect: _____

SPECIAL AREAS

- Eyes: _____
- Lips: _____
- Neck and chest: _____

On each line, write down the products or ingredients that you're looking for. For example, after "Cleanse," be sure to note "nonsoap." Then decide if you'd prefer an exfoliating or a moisturizing cleanser. After "Exfoliate," you might indicate whether you want a chemical exfoliant, such as glycolic acid or salicylic acid, or a physical exfoliant, such as microdermabrasion particles or a Buf-Puf.

You might consider combining "Moisturize" and "Rejuvenate," with an eye toward finding a product that will both hydrate and reduce lines. If you are a heavy smoker with especially prominent lip lines, I'd suggest investing in neuropeptide for around your lips—and certainly a peptide for your entire face.

As for "Protect," remember my preference for zinc. That

said, try to get a sample of a zinc-based sunscreen, so you can test it to be sure that you like it—and will use it.

The "Special Areas" section is for your Uninvited Elements (UEs). For instance, if you're bothered by undereye puffiness or dark circles, now is the time to investigate products that might minimize or eliminate these UEs. Prone to dry lips? Note that here. Age spots or discoloration on your chest? Ditto.

Do one more sweep of your bathroom sink, medicine cabinet, vanity, and purse—as well as your piles of Essentials and Not-Sures. You may already have some products with the necessary ingredients. In that case, you might decide to stick with, for example, your current facial cleanser (provided it's nonsoap) and sunscreen, and put that money toward a hydroquinone product to help fade those age spots on your chest.

Now . . . it's time to buy!

STOCKING UP

Some Beauty Campers may need just one or two new skin-care products. Others might be starting from scratch, putting together an entirely new regimen. No matter which group you fall into, you now have the knowledge to navigate the skin-care aisles and cosmetics counters with ease.

Again, I encourage you to take this book with you when you go shopping. You may need to sneak a peek at My Favorite Ingredients in Week #2 or the Survival Basics above. Eventually, all of the ingredients will be well known to you—and brand names, too. For now, though, play it safe and keep a reference at hand.

Just as when you went on your exploratory mission, remember

to try every skin-care product before making a purchase. If you aren't sure about a particular product, see if you can get an amply sized sample. If you're dying to try something expensive, like a peptide, perhaps a few fellow Beauty Campers—or your sisters or a group of friends—would be willing to invest in a jar to share with you. Be sure to buy the smallest available quantities to start.

If you're like most women, you may not go out without at least a hint of makeup on your face. This can get a little tricky when sampling products. Instead of applying them on top of makeup, use the skin on your inner arm or in the crease of your elbow. It's much like the skin on your face. Likewise, if you want to test an eye cream, apply it to your neck, which is most similar to the delicate skin around your eyes.

As you select your products, keep close tabs on your budget. You can find great skin-care products in every price range, so think twice before spending a lot on a high-end brand. For example, a good-quality glycolic acid or salicylic acid cleanser should be fairly inexpensive. What you save on the cleanser could be put toward a pricier product, like a peptide.

A word of caution to any Gung Ho Campers out there: Please, please exercise restraint while on your skin-care shopping excursions. You may be prone to buying products the same way some women buy shoes: on impulse. So make a pact with yourself or another Gung Ho type to put an end to this mindless consumption. Don't return home with a shopping bag brimming with products.

Remember, too, to read those product labels. And watch out for the Poison Ivy ingredients!

CAMP ACTIVITY #4
SHOW AND TELL

Once you start using your new products, you should notice a difference in your skin relatively quickly. For instance, peptides have been known to improve skin after just one use. Are you seeing any changes or improvement?

Now for the real test: It's time to dig out that digital camera or Polaroid once again. You're going to take several pictures of your face—without makeup, in good lighting, and from the same angles as your Orientation photos. These are your first "after" photos, taken just days into your new skin-care regimen.

Compare your new photos with your Orientation photos. Is there a visible difference in your skin? If not, perhaps the improvements are too minor to detect just yet. You may want to glue or tape your new photos on the designated pages at the back of this book, so you'll have them for future reference.

Now let's discuss your skin-care purchases. Obviously, cosmetics companies invest lots of time and money developing products that feel and smell good. They even employ human testers to help assess the desirability (and marketability) of a particular product. But everyone is different—what appeals to one person may turn off another.

As you survey your new skin-care products, ask yourself the following questions.

1. Which nonsoap cleanser did you decide to try?

2. Does your face feel cleaner or a bit too dry?

3. How does the exfoliant feel on your skin—too strong or just right?

4. Does your moisturizer feel sticky or just right?

5. How about your sunscreen—sticky or just right?

6. Do you still like the smell of everything?

7. How does your skin look—any reactions yet?

8. Does your makeup go on smoothly over the products you use in the morning?

If you are sharing products with other Beauty Campers, arrive at this week's meeting with your new products and a bag of empty travel-size containers so everyone can swap and sample. Discuss how you went about choosing your products from all the options out there. How many campers actually read the ingredient lists? How much did each camper spend? Was anyone tempted to go over budget? No fudging!

After the first week of using the basic skin-care regimen that I've outlined, you really should see a modicum of improvement in your skin. And it should be unique improvement—something that hasn't occurred with other (cheaper or weaker) products that you've tried. In other words, the moisturizer that cost $100 shouldn't do what a jar of Eucerin cream, at $10, can do. It ought to perform significantly better!

That said, be patient. Your new skin-care regimen could be incredibly effective at restoring your skin's appearance. But it may be about 4 weeks before you see truly dramatic results. Please give your products a chance to work before running off to a doctor's office and begging for Botox.

SCARY CAMP STORY:
AN AT-HOME PEEL GONE AWRY

As you may have guessed, my daughters love to treat their own skin—and sometimes they can get a little carried away. (Please don't say they take after me!)

Today Katrina is a wonderfully responsible undergrad. When she was 14, though, she decided to leave on an at-home glycolic acid peel that is meant to be washed off after 10 to 20 minutes. She'd gotten good results with a similar but milder product, and she figured that "more is better."

Unfortunately, instead of producing even better results, the peel started to really hurt after about 40 minutes. Katrina washed it off—but 20 to 30 minutes too late. She was left with what looked like a bad sunburn on some parts of her face. Within a day, she was getting scabs in the creases around her nose. I rushed to her aid with a 1 percent (over-the-counter) hydrocortisone cream, but the scabs lasted for 5 days.

The good news: She never did anything like that again—and she learned the importance of following the label directions. They exist for a reason!

EXTREME CHALLENGE
RETINOL

The Extreme Challenges aren't for everybody. But if you just can't wait to eliminate those creases, crow's-feet, and other facial lines, you may want to try a retinol product. A milder relative of Retin-A, retinol has proven effective in reducing the depth—and therefore the appearance—of fine lines and some grooves.

These days, many drugstore brands contain retinol. If you go this route, be prepared to fine-tune how you use the product—especially if you have sensitive skin. For myself, as much as I like retinol and as effective as it is in reducing lines and evening skin tone, I've never been able to tolerate using a 0.3 percent product more often than every 2 or 3 days.

I suggest trying a mild retinol formula to start, following the label directions. Pay attention to any redness or dryness; it might feel as though you have a mild sunburn. In that case, cut back your applications to just once or twice a week.

On the other hand, if you already are using other physician-strength formulations, you may want to try a retinol product from a dermatologist's line. Some of these products can be 10 or more times stronger than store brands.

EXTREME CHALLENGE
NEUROPEPTIDES

Neuropeptides can reduce the appearance of dynamic lines for some people. They also happen to be very expensive, compared with other skin-care products. A jar of Freeze 24/7, which the manufacturer markets as "a safe alternative to Botox," sells for $115. You don't want to drop that much money on a neuropeptide only to discover that it doesn't work for you—or that a cheaper product works just as well.

This is a situation where buddying up with two or three other Beauty Campers could come in handy. You could split

The Half-Face Test

If you're not convinced that your new skin-care products are working, you can do what I call the half-face test. Imagine a line running down the center of your face. Use your new regimen on one side of the line, while continuing with your old products on the other side. Just be consistent about which products go on which side. You might label your products *R* (right side) and *L* (left side) to help keep them straight.

The half-face test also is a good tool for comparing highly priced products with their less expensive counterparts. For example, if you're among a group of Beauty Campers, you might chip in for an expensive cream from an upscale department store. Then try it in a half-face test against a cheaper product from the drugstore.

I use the half-face test in clinical trials of my own skin-care line. No new formulation is considered effective unless it produces significant improvement on the side of the face to which it is applied.

the cost of a jar of Freeze 24/7, plus a jar of DermaFreeze 365, which sells for about $39 in drugstores. Both products contain GABA complex, one of the very popular neuropeptide ingredients. You can pit the two against each other in a half-face test. (For instructions, see above.)

CAMP LESSON
FINE-TUNING YOUR REGIMEN

Fine-tuning your skin-care regimen is an essential part of getting it right. You need to pay attention to how the ingredients are performing and your skin is reacting. You also need to be sensitive to your own level of motivation. Is this regimen really practical for your lifestyle and body clock?

For example, if you find yourself too sleepy at bedtime to adequately cleanse your face and apply any nighttime products, then you might consider doing it earlier—say, an hour or two after dinner. There's no hard-and-fast rule that you must wait until immediately before you go to bed.

Occasionally skipping your nighttime regimen—or wanting to—is understandable to me, given how hectic our lives can be and how exhausted we are by day's end. Your morning regimen is a different story. You should be waking up well rested (especially if you're getting 30 extra minutes of sleep, as I recommend), with enough time to run through all of your skin-care steps. If that isn't the case, I suggest the following: Before going to bed, lay out all of the products that you'll need the next morning. That way, they're waiting for you when you roll out of bed. I got into this habit myself a few years ago. Now I need just 2 minutes to run through my entire A.M. skin-care routine.

Something else that might help to get you on track in the morning: Keep all of your necessary products on a wicker tray next to your bathroom sink or on a side counter. Most products are not that temperature sensitive and will remain effective as long as they are kept away from a hot radiator or a cold window. Some of us waste time just trying to find our products and then, when we're done with them, returning them to a less-than-practical location. Also, if you happen to misplace a product, you might completely forget to use it. Out of sight, out of mind!

Having said all this, if you do happen to miss your skin-care regimen one morning or evening, believe me, it isn't the end of the world. But do try to get back on track as soon as possible. Otherwise, you won't know for certain whether or not what you're doing is working—especially while you still are experimenting with products. What's the point of the expense and effort if you can't get a truly accurate assessment of the results?

Other situations will arise that may require you to make adjustments in your skin-care regimen. For example, climate changes make a dramatic difference in your skin; what works in summer might need fine-tuning in autumn and then again in winter. This is particularly true if you live in a harsher climate or spend a great deal of time outdoors.

Climate changes happen more abruptly, of course, when you travel. If you are going to a warm-weather climate, expect your skin to be less dry. But the warmer temperatures also may aggravate a tendency to break out. If you're acne prone, you may want to purchase a salicylic acid cleanser for a trip like this. And for Beauty Campers who battle frizzy hair in humid climates, a good leave-in conditioner should help keep it under control. (We'll talk more about hair care in Week #5.)

On the other hand, if you're going on a ski trip, the best skin-care survival strategy is to invest in a very moisturizing sunscreen—ideally, a sports formulation. This strategy also applies for travel to higher altitudes, where the combination of sun and dry air can do a number on your skin. This can be especially rough if your skin is prone to redness or flaking to begin with.

Some Beauty Campers tend to break out when they travel, regardless of climate considerations. It's the stress, the jet lag, the changing sleep schedule, even the food that we so often end up eating when we're in a rush. If you have a tendency to break out while on the road, pack a salicylic acid cleanser or another salicylic acid product to tend to acne flare-ups—and maybe a hydrating calming mask with camphor, cucumber, or chamomile.

Beyond travel, your exercise program is—or should be—a factor in your skin-care regimen. For example, if you start your day with a run or another workout, you really don't need to cleanse your face first. As a Beauty Camper, you will have applied all those terrific products the evening before. Simply dab your face with tepid water and apply a good waterproof sunscreen—one that won't run or sting your eyes. (The sports formulas made by Coppertone and Neutrogena claim to not sting.) You can do your daily skin-care regimen after your shower.

If you're a swimmer, you might want to apply a waterproof, zinc-based sunscreen before heading into the pool—even if it's indoors. The zinc has the added benefit of calming and protecting the skin from the effects of chlorine. I must say, though, that I am amazed by how few of my patients seem to be irritated by chlorine, which sometimes can be overdone. For myself, I love to use a soothing mask after a day of swimming.

When to Call It Quits

Suppose you're on day 3 or week 5 of your new skin-care regimen and you suddenly notice that a certain product doesn't feel good on your skin. Listen to your body! Any dryness, redness, or irritation is your cue to discontinue the product for several days. You can try it again once your symptoms subside, but this time, use it less frequently. I have products in my regimen that I use only two or three times a week, not every day.

Likewise, if a product stings on application, I suggest cutting back on how often you apply it. If the label directions say twice a day, go to just once a day. Please bear in mind the distinction between "tingling" and "stinging." If a product makes your skin tingle, it probably is doing some good. If it truly stings or burns, then it may be too strong for you.

You don't need to stick with any product that is causing a reaction. If you weren't so sure about its benefits in the first place, you should feel free to permanently remove it from your skin-care regimen. Perhaps you can trade products with a fellow Beauty Camper. She may have something in her regimen that isn't right for her but is perfect for you.

Week #3 Review

- *Create a skin-care regimen that works with your personality, not against it.*
- *Purchase products based on ingredients rather than marketing campaigns.*
- *Remember the five Survival Basics: Cleansing, exfoliating, moisturizing, rejuvenating, and protecting.*

- *Fine-tune your regimen as necessary. You may need to keep testing products until you find just the right ones for your skin. How many women marry the first person they date?*
- *Don't throw out the baby with the bathwater. If you like a product but it irritates your skin, simply cut back on the frequency of application. You might also pair the product with a calming agent—for example, follow a glycolic acid peel with a soothing chamomile cleanser.*
- *I hope you've gotten that good, soft pillowcase.*
- *How are the facial exercises going?*
- *Now get some sleep!*

Week #4

Your Skin Tone

This week's agenda: Clearing your skin of age spots, brown patches, dark circles, broken blood vessels, and areas of redness, discoloration, and uneven pigment

We focus on our facial lines and grooves because we're a youth-obsessed culture. Some of us are certain that with a smooth face, like that of a department-store mannequin, we'd look so much younger and better. But would we?

I, for one, am not so sure. I love my smile lines, which really are a little more like grooves, off to the sides of my mouth. They've been there since my twenties—and I plan to die with them, too. Smoothness can be overrated. Certain lines and wrinkles give us uniqueness and make a face seem warm and endearing.

Not that I haven't tried to keep my own wrinkles under control. But sometimes I wish our culture and my patients paid more attention to skin tone. That's where I notice the most Uninvited Elements (UEs) of all. For example, I've never met an age spot that I liked—or seen one that gave someone's face a bit of character.

Actually, "age spots" is something of a misnomer, as even twentysomethings can get them. Perhaps a few are lurking on your face or body, with dozens more waiting to appear. The funny thing is how common they are, yet how offended my patients can be when I tell them that those new "freckles" really are burgeoning *solar lentigos*, the medical term for what most of us describe as an age spot or liver spot. My patients take the news so personally. It's as though I'm telling them that they have hemorrhoids.

But Beauty Camp is about honesty—and when it comes to skin tone, we need to be honest with ourselves. Our faces may be blotchier than they once were, smattered with freckles, red or scaly patches, raised brown *seborrheic keratoses*—and, yes, age spots! We have more moles than ever, more warts and small cystic growths, and more broken capillaries and blood vessels. We have dark circles. Red noses! Stains! Even if every line and groove were to disappear from our faces, these UEs would keep our skin from looking its healthy, vibrant best.

I don't mean to harp on what may be a sore subject, but most of the wear and tear that shows in a woman's face as she grows older starts during her youthful days in the sun. If you've gotten through the past decade—during which the medical community and the media have made every effort to educate the public about the effects of excessive sun exposure on the skin—and you still believe you don't need sun protection . . . well, maybe I can't change your mind, either. But I surely will try.

Let me say, briefly, that in addition to three kinds of skin cancer, photoaging—the product of sun exposure plus time—is responsible for most of the UEs that you may be noticing in your face now. These include not just wrinkles but also age spots; brown splotches; "chicken skin" (the yellowish hue that can appear around the eyes and in other areas); broken capillaries; dryness; cracking; sagging; and networks of red, brown, and white patches on the neck and chest (not to mention porcelain white patches on the arms and legs).

I know, I know. We can't do much now about our glory days of overexposure. But at the very least, we can admit to our past follies—and acknowledge the present consequences. If you spent any amount of time outdoors in your childhood and young adulthood, you probably have visible signs of sun damage on your face. Now is the time to deal with them.

CAMP ACTIVITY #1
OH, THOSE WAYWARD SPOTS

Please take a mirror and look at your face in very bright light. It could be outdoors on a sunny day or under the harsh fluorescent lighting of your workplace. Do you see even the tiniest brown patches? If so, please don't resist the thought that you are developing age spots. Once a Beauty Camper admits to them and goes hunting for them, she can begin getting rid of them. Fading existing age spots and preventing new ones are natural outcomes of practicing good skin care on a daily basis.

As its medical name—solar lentigo—suggests, an age spot truly is the result of the sun. You will notice more age spots on the sun-exposed areas of your face, neck, chest, arms, and hands. (They have nothing to do with liver disease, by the way. I think the name "liver spot" comes from their looking, at their worst, like a piece of liver on the skin surface.)

Generally, age spots are rare in women under age 30—though in my own practice, I'm seeing more women in their twenties with them, usually as the result of too much time spent in tanning parlors. Once the spots start coming, they keep coming . . . and coming. One year you'll notice just three or four. The next year, you'll notice more.

Out, Darned Spot!

Everybody's skin is a little different. Some women can completely erase their age spots with an at-home preparation. Others will notice some fading but not a complete cure. As a rule, I recommend trying at-home treatments first. (We'll explore in-office treatment options in Camp Activity #2.)

Among the effective remedies for age spots are two skin-care ingredients that by now should be very familiar to you: glycolic acid and retinol. Beyond reducing the appearance of lines and grooves, they're known to fade age spots and other skin discolorations, too. I don't mean to suggest that all age spots will go away completely with regular use of these acidic concoctions. But if you've noticed improvement—that is, fading of your spots—since you've added glycolic acid or retinol to your basic skin-care regimen, then by all means proceed with your product of choice.

If you're using glycolic acid, you can continue to apply it to your entire face. If you're using retinol—or Retin-A in any form—you might try dabbing the solution on your age spots more frequently than you are using it on the rest of your face. Applying retinol to your entire face on a daily basis probably would irritate your skin, but concentrating the solution right on a spot just might do the trick.

If you're not seeing any change in your age spots with glycolic acid or retinol, then it's time to bring in a good fade cream. These products are designed specifically to even skin tone and lighten any discoloration. The best ingredient in a fade cream is hydroquinone (HQ), a chemical that prevents skin cells from making excess pigment. There are other fade ingredients on the market—things like gooseberry extract, kojic acid, and licorice. But based on the clinical test results that I've seen, HQ consistently seems to perform better.

With HQ, as with certain other skin-care ingredients, you can get too much of a good thing. Recently I saw two different women who had been applying prescription-strength HQ, sandwiched between layers of moisturizer, before bed. This caused pretty severe irritation. I advised both patients to switch to an over-the-counter (2 percent) hydrocortisone cream and use it twice a day. The results were spectacular. When one of the women came back for follow-up 2 weeks later, I didn't recognize her—that's how much better she looked. She told me that she actually had been in some pain from the extreme irritation of the concentrated HQ. Once she revised her regimen, several of her friends commented that her skin looked years younger—and her smile helped, too!

Most of my patients find that using a 2 percent HQ formulation twice a day is effective at fading age spots. You should be able to find a 2 percent product in a drugstore or online. Contrary to common sense, it's best to apply it all over your face, not just on your age spots. The ingredient works in any area where excess pigment is being made, so by applying it all over, you'll not only fade spots that are visible but also prevent those that aren't apparent to the naked eye or with a magnifying mirror . . . yet.

To enhance the effectiveness of HQ, you might pair it with glycolic acid—ideally, a physician-strength formula. For simplicity's sake, some products combine these two ingredients—usually, 2 percent HQ with 5 to 15 percent glycolic acid. Again, such a product would go on the entire face.

In my 25 years of dermatologic practice, I've found that the one-two punch of HQ and glycolic acid works as well as prescription-strength HQ for more than 90 percent of my patients. It has worked for me, too. Recently I was trying on a dress when my daughter Katrina walked in. She said, "You know, Mom, I remember seeing an old photo of you with your chest covered in age spots." Ten years later, all the spots are gone. Not bad!

This brings me to a very important point about age spots:

Maintenance, Maintenance, Maintenance

A common mistake in treating age spots and other skin discolorations is abandoning treatment once you look better. But this is a little like quitting antibiotics as soon as you feel better. Neither is a good idea. Since the sun exposure that caused the spots most likely occurred decades ago, your skin essentially has been programmed to start making new spots once you stop treatment. And it will.

That said, once you've been using a hydroquinone (HQ) product for 2 months and any age spots have faded or vanished to your satisfaction, your best bet is to slowly wean yourself off treatment. Apply HQ just once a day instead of twice. After 2 weeks, cut back further to three times a week. After another month, stop using HQ altogether. Wait 2 months, then resume treatment.

There's a good reason for this strategy: Constant use of HQ can cause you to become allergic to it. And the sticky thing about an HQ allergy is that your skin may darken as a symptom of your reaction.

One other note: Even while you're stepping off hydroquinone, continue to protect your face with sunscreen. Your skin will be more sun-sensitive from treatment.

We all know women who've apparently been vigilant about preventing spots on their faces but haven't paid nearly as much attention to their chest and hands. It's a bit disturbing, really—as though their youthful faces are attached to older bodies. This is why I suggest using these remedies that we've discussed here not only on your face but also on other sun-exposed areas—particularly the tops of your hands and below your collarbones.

Generally, if your spots are going to clear from the HQ/glycolic acid treatment, you should see dramatic improvement within 6 to 8 weeks. If that doesn't happen, you probably need to pursue another course of action—either asking your dermatologist for a prescription-strength (3 percent or higher) HQ preparation or investigating in-office treatments.

Maybe It's Not What You Think

While you were examining your face in the mirror, you may have found other kinds of discolorations that didn't seem exactly like age spots. And you could be right. There are several kinds of spots and stains, and dermatologists make distinctions between them. Many of the effective remedies for fading or erasing these UEs are the same. Still, you will need to determine which kind of discoloration you have to be sure you're treating it properly.

Besides age spots, the most common discolorations in facial skin are melasma, postinflammatory hyperpigmentation, and seborrheic keratoses. I'll explain each of them here, hopefully in enough detail that you'll be able to identify which you've got. We'll talk about effective at-home treatments, too. (We'll cover in-office treatments in just a bit.)

Melasma: This masklike stain looks like a faint shadow on the skin. Sometimes it affects the upper lip, creating the appearance of a "mustache" of dark pigment.

Some women are born with a predisposition to melasma. Though sun exposure can trigger the condition, hormones also play a big role. It is most likely to affect women during pregnancy or while they're on hormone replacement therapy (HRT) or oral contraceptives. If you develop a bad case of melasma while you're pregnant, it could recur if you begin HRT or oral contraceptives later on.

The at-home treatment for melasma is the same as for age spots. Be aware that if HRT or an oral contraceptive is the cause of the problem, it may not resolve until you stop your medication (after consulting your prescribing physician, of course).

Do not use hydroquinone to treat melasma while you are pregnant. For several of my patients, combining a strong sunscreen with micronized zinc oxide—one of three ingredients that block the sun's harmful UVA rays—improved the skin's appearance during pregnancy.

Postinflammatory hyperpigmentation: This is the medical term for dark spots that tend to occur after a serious or chronic insult to the skin, such as a kitchen burn, an insect bite, or a severe acne breakout. Though sun exposure raises the risk of these spots, they are most common in people with a genetic predisposition to skin staining—particularly those of Mediterranean, Middle Eastern, or African heritage.

I know this from personal experience. I am Italian, with light skin. If I happen to sustain an injury—say, by burning myself while cooking—a dark spot will appear at the site of the injury within days and could last for months if I don't treat it.

Sometimes the spot is preceded by redness, which can linger for days or even weeks before giving way to brown.

The best approach to treating postinflammatory hyperpigmentation, if you are susceptible to it as I am, is to be proactive. Immediately apply hydrocortisone cream to burns, bug bites, and other injuries that leave your skin vulnerable to staining. Ideally, you'll be able to start treatment at the first sign of redness, before any brown appears. You won't get the staining that occurs in the postinflammatory stage if you clear up the inflammation (redness) first.

In the case of a bug bite, I suggest applying hydrocortisone cream two or three times daily, beginning as soon as possible after the bite. The cream will not only promote healing, but also alleviate itching and other symptoms that may cause you to pick at the bite—further raising your risk of staining. If bugs seem intent on making a meal out of you, be extra vigilant about using insect repellent before heading outdoors.

If you miss your window of opportunity to begin treatment and notice a dark spot at the site of the injury, it's a good idea to add topical hydrocortisone to the HQ/glycolic acid combination that we discussed for age spots. In my experience, any staining—even if it is several years old—will improve much faster with twice-daily hydrocortisone applications in conjunction with the HQ/glycolic acid preparation.

Please take care not to use products that are too harsh for your skin, because they can aggravate staining rather than helping to clear it. I recommend starting with an over-the-counter 2 percent HQ cream, along with a gentle glycolic acid fade cream. The results can be quite dramatic. (This regimen works quite well for acne scarring, too.)

How long before you see results? It depends on how long you had the dark spot when you began treatment. Beauty Campers need to temper their expectations with patience when treating this kind of problem. If you don't see some improvement within 6 weeks, I suggest consulting a dermatologist, who can assess the problem and discuss further treatment options.

Seborrheic keratoses: These raised brown spots may look like patches of darker pigment, but in fact, they are benign (non-cancerous) growths on the skin. They are hereditary, which means you've done nothing to cause them. Unfortunately, it also means you can't do anything to keep new ones from forming.

One particular variety of seborrheic keratosis is nearly flat; it can be reduced, if not almost eliminated, with a strong glycolic acid formulation. Otherwise, these growths need to be removed by a physician.

EXTREME CHALLENGE
IS IT WORKING?

Treating long-standing age spots and other discolorations can feel a little like trying to lose those last stubborn 10 pounds. If you don't see any signs of progress, you may wonder if what you're doing is having any effect at all.

Should you find yourself in this predicament, one easy solution is to take a few photos of your face at various angles under bright (but not too bright) light. Then, with a red pen or marker, circle on the photo any spots, patches, stains, and other discolorations that you see. This way you have a record of their size and intensity. Take another set of photos in a week and again in 2 weeks. Compare the new shots with the older ones; do you see any changes in your skin?

Another option is what I call the half-face test, which we discussed in Week #3. To recap: Apply the treatment to one side of your face but not the other. After about a week, compare the two sides. Once you're satisfied that the treatment is working, by all means start using it on your entire face.

CAMP ACTIVITY #2
INVESTIGATING THE NEXT STEP

If you've not been seeing a dermatologist on a regular basis, the prospect of scheduling an appointment to discuss in-office skin treatments may be rather daunting. Some patients feel overwhelmed, out of their depth, powerless. They do nothing but surrender and hope for the best.

Going to a dermatologist—or any doctor, for that matter—should never be a mindless leap of faith. I'm not saying so because I went to medical school, and I haven't felt intimidated by other doctors and their expertise. I have. It's just that all of us could do a better job of arming ourselves with knowledge so we feel more confident about the skin-care decisions we make. As with most things in life, a little research into in-office treatments can go a long way.

In this day and age, it's almost impossible not to hear stories about the miraculous results of laser therapy, photofacials, and glycolic acid peels. Our friends may have had very good experiences with these treatments—or very bad ones. To make sure you don't wind up disappointed (or looking worse), it's important to find the right doctor and the right procedure. With such an abundance of methods for treating age spots and other skin discolorations, you'll want to choose one that is effective and low risk and won't break your budget.

Perhaps you already have a dermatologist whom you trust and could consult about treatment options. I suggest making a call to his or her office and asking the questions below before making an appointment. If you don't have a dermatologist, you'll need to find one. Your family doctor or the physician referral service of your local hospital can provide leads. So, too, can family members and friends, as well as other Beauty Campers. Also check online; for example, the American Academy of Dermatology Web site (www.aad.org) allows you to search for board-certified dermatologists in your area.

Once you've identified a few candidates, start making phone calls. Remember, you aren't scheduling an appointment just yet: You're on a fact-finding mission. If the receptionist can't answer your questions—or seems overly eager to book you for a consultation—ask to speak with a nurse or medical assistant. Your call shouldn't take more than a few minutes of this person's time. If he or she resists providing answers over the phone, it may be your cue to move on. You need this information to make a good decision about your treatment. Among the questions you should ask a current or prospective dermatologist:

- Does this doctor treat age spots and other skin discolorations? (If not, keep shopping around.)
- Which procedures does he or she offer, and what type of equipment does he or she use? (We'll explore your options in detail below.)

- Are the procedures or machines new? (The newer they are, the less experience the doctor will have with them.)
- Does the doctor perform the procedures, or could that be left to someone else?
- Has the doctor (or his or her associate) received appropriate training in these procedures and equipment? How many of the procedures has the doctor performed?
- What is the worst possible outcome of each treatment in question?
- What is the approximate cost of the treatments?
- Would any of the treatments be covered by health insurance? (Probably not, for treatments that are largely cosmetic.)
- When is the next available appointment? (In metropolitan areas, many dermatologists are so deluged with patients that the next available appointment is 2 months away.)

Do thank the nurse or medical assistant for taking time to address your questions, and mention that once you've been able to thoroughly review the information, you may call back to schedule an appointment. Please don't commit until you've contacted the rest of the doctors' offices on your list.

The fact is, while a certain doctor might seem top-notch on paper and his or her staff may be very obliging over the phone, your objective is to find someone who is skilled in the procedures and equipment you require. I know it might seem that all dermatologists provide pretty much the same services and use pretty much the same equipment, but it isn't so. A doctor might simply offer what's available to him or her at the moment. That isn't good enough.

With all this in mind, let's take a look at the more common in-office treatments—spot by spot, stain by stain. Along the way, I'll offer my own insights and advice, based on my experience as a dermatologist—and as my own favorite guinea pig!

In-Office Treatments for Age Spots

For age spots, a favorite treatment among dermatologists is what's known as a *glycolic acid peel* or *glycolic wash*. It involves applying a 70 percent glycolic acid formulation (as opposed to the 10 percent formulations dispensed for at-home use) to an entire anatomical area—face, neck, chest, and/or hands—not just to the spots. Usually a course of treatment consists of 6 to 10 peels spaced 1 to 2 weeks apart.

I've found this treatment to be helpful both in fading existing spots and discouraging new ones from forming. Each application costs roughly $50 to $75; an entire series can run from $350 to $600, depending on where you live. (The advantage of living in a metropolitan area is that you probably have access to the very latest skin treatments. But you could pay premium prices for them, too.)

If you have particularly stubborn age spots that don't go away after a series of glycolic acid peels, your doctor might choose to test-treat a few of the spots with a stronger preparation called *trichloroacetic acid* (TCA). I suggest that you and your doctor wait at least 12 weeks before deciding if TCA is a good approach for fading any remaining stubborn spots, since spot-by-spot applications may leave you with slightly darker patches for 2 or 3 months. Treatment with TCA runs from $200 to $300.

Another heavily marketed treatment for stubborn age spots

is *laser therapy*. There are several types of lasers, with varying brand names. What's important to remember here is that laser therapy involves a controlled burning of the skin. It is very damaging to skin cells. I have several patients who had gone to other doctors for treatment of tiny brown solar lentigos, only to end up with permanent, bigger, darker brown patches than they'd had originally. Their doctors treated larger areas than necessary and used lasers that burned the skin badly. Unfortunately, these people ended up worse off instead of better.

This is why I recommend a very conservative approach with laser therapy. Ask your doctor to test-treat a spot or two, then wait 3 months. At your follow-up, the two of you can assess how the treatment has affected your skin and decide whether you want to continue with the same laser, try a different one—or switch to a completely different therapy.

My personal favorite in-office treatment for age spots, as well as for overall facial rejuvenation, is *intense pulsed light* (IPL). Unlike a laser, which is a steady, focused light beam, the IPL is more like a flashbulb continuously going off. (For this reason, many doctors refer to IPL treatments as photofacials.)

IPL is fast becoming more popular than the laser. Why? Because when administering an IPL treatment, doctors generally run the light beam over the entire face. Therefore, you'll see greater overall improvement in the quality of your skin for the time and money that you invest.

But Beauty Campers need to be aware that not all doctors have an IPL machine. I urge you, once again, to be a smart consumer. Ask specifically whether your doctor has access to an IPL machine. In the best-case scenario, if your doctor doesn't have access to an IPL—or to any other machine that would be beneficial to your skin—then he or she will send you elsewhere. But in today's marketplace, this doesn't always happen.

IPL has proven to be great at removing age spots from the face, chest, and hands. The spots will become darker right after treatment, then start dropping off in 4 to 7 days—though you may not see results as quickly on the chest and hands as on the face. IPL is also good for clearing a red flush from the chest. (We'll talk more about redness shortly.) There's no recovery period to speak of, making IPL treatments virtually risk free.

If the treatments have a downside, it's that they must be done as a series—usually three to five sessions spaced about 2 to 4 weeks apart. The average cost for three sessions is $1,200, but that's still much less than laser therapy. A laser can be very expensive, especially if it's used extensively in one area. Doctors often charge per pulse of the laser, which means that someone with many age spots could spend thousands of dollars to completely clear their skin.

Be aware that some doctors like to intensify IPL treatments by applying Levulan, a light-sensitizing solution, to a patient's skin 30 to 60 minutes beforehand. Levulan preconditions the skin to the light source, producing a much more intense reaction. Sometimes scabbing occurs.

While combining IPL with Levulan can yield dramatic results, it also can increase discomfort from treatment and extend healing time. In my opinion, IPL alone is a much better choice, because you can get great results with minimal discomfort.

SCARY CAMP STORY:
AN EXCEPTION TO EVERY RULE!

If you experience a sudden onslaught of brown patches that appear over a period of days to a week, they probably are not simple age spots but, rather, a sign of a more obscure condition called *berloque dermatitis*. It is a form of sun sensitivity brought on by contact with limes or lemons.

Berloque dermatitis can affect anyone at any age, even teenagers. It seems more likely to occur in warm weather, when people head outside for picnics, parties, and other outdoor events. Someone may drink a beverage with lemon or lime squeezed into it, only to end up with multiple frecklelike stains on the forearms and backs of the hands.

The standard treatment for berloque dermatitis is a mild hydrocortisone cream plus over-the-counter-strength hydroquinone. Generally speaking, the stains clear up almost as quickly as they appear. But after one bout of berloque dermatitis, you need to be extra careful to never allow your skin to come in contact with lime or lemon juice again. You could get new stains every time.

In-Office Treatment for Melasma

Many of the in-office treatments for age spots will be effective for melasma as well. A glycolic acid peel—the most gentle to the skin—is a good starting point, since people who are prone to pigment problems could experience an adverse reaction to a stronger therapy. If you develop melasma during pregnancy, I would encourage you to wait a while before seeking treatment. Sometimes the condition resolves, with just the use of the right sunscreen, within 3 to 6 months of having a baby or coming off of oral contraceptives.

In-Office Treatment for Post inflammatory Hyperpigmentation

In general, in-office treatments aren't all that effective for fading this type of staining. That said, a series of light salicylic acid peels—even just two or three—can make a difference, especially in combination with any at-home treatment that you already have begun. By exfoliating your skin, the peels allow for better penetration of topical preparations. The cost of a single salicylic acid peel is in the range of $120 to $150.

In-Office Treatment for Sebhorreic Keratoses

The simplest in-office treatment for sebhorreic keratoses is *light electrodessication.* In other words, a doctor burns off the spots with a cauterizing machine, one of the most time-honored therapies in dermatology. I always tell my patients to prepare for the smell of burning skin—their own. (Of course, what I'm burning off is something that they didn't want on their skin in the first place.)

While use of a cauterizing machine is necessary to remove sebhorreic keratoses, a too-high setting may leave behind some scarring. I prefer to start by test-treating one or two lesions at a low setting. The patient returns for follow-up 3 or 4 weeks later. If the keratoses are gone, I will treat the rest of the lesions at the same low setting as on the initial visit. If I don't see good resolution of the lesions, I will slightly increase the power on the instrument and again treat just one or two spots. I'll proceed in this way until eventually I find just the right setting for this particular patient.

The price of electrodessication can run from $150 to $300, depending on the individual office fee and the number of lesions requiring treatment.

CAMP ACTIVITY #3
REDUCE THE RED

Sip a steaming cup of green tea or a glass of red wine, or have a bowl of hot soup or a package of spicy wasabi crackers. After 15 minutes, wander into your well-lit bathroom and look in the mirror. Is your nose red? Are your cheeks flushed? Are you starting to look like Bill Clinton after a jog?

By our mid-thirties, many of us routinely develop a red flush in our faces after we consume something hot, spicy, or alcoholic. The flush is typical of *rosacea*, a form of adult acne (though not every woman who's prone to redness and flushing has rosacea, as we soon will see).

Fully manifested, rosacea has three components: an acne breakout that runs down the center of the face and involves the forehead, nose, and central cheeks and chin; redness and broken blood vessels that resemble a sunburn; and, in the most extreme cases, a condition called *rhinophyma*, or bulbous swelling of the nose.

The good news about rosacea is that it responds very well to the antibiotic tetracycline. Even someone who's had the condition for a long time will see a remarkable clearing—sometimes after just a few days—once she is properly diagnosed and prescribed tetracycline.

The bad news is that because rosacea is a chronic skin condition, many women who have it end up going on and off antibiotics for years. This can be troublesome, as repeated use of antibiotics may promote vaginal yeast infections, among other things. Worse, many diagnosed cases of rosacea aren't rosacea at all, so some women may be taking antibiotics needlessly and at the expense of their future health. In fact, one study suggests that women who take antibiotics for more than 1,000 days of their lives are at higher risk for breast cancer.

If you truly have rosacea, you can take steps to reduce the likelihood of a flare-up. One is to clear your diet of potential triggers such as hot beverages, spicy foods, and alcohol—especially red wine. I have a mild case of rosacea myself, and if I drink just a single glass of wine, I can get pimples that last for several days.

If you're on a maintenance regimen of antibiotics, you might talk with your doctor about reducing your dosage. For instance, many of my patients with rosacea are able to remain clear and recurrence free if they take a minimum amount of tetracycline. Some require just one pill a week.

There are topical treatments for rosacea. The most time-tested are MetroCream and MetroGel, both of which have proven to be very effective. They greatly reduce the likelihood of a recurrence and may keep some people from having to go back on tetracycline.

Among the newer topical treatments for rosacea are the prescription preparations Plexion, Rosac, and Finacea. Since people who have rosacea may become resistant to a particular treatment over time, it is a good idea to switch creams every 6 to 12 months for best results.

Okay. Now that we've gotten the scary stuff out of the way, let's face the facts about redness and facial flushing. The vast majority of cases are caused not by rosacea but, rather, by one of these two things.

- Hormonal fluctuations that begin well before menopause, usually by our late thirties
- An irritant with which our faces have come into contact—bar soap, fragrance, detergent, fabric softener, or something else

Let's examine each of these factors in turn.

Redness Caused by Fluctuating Hormones

If hormones are to blame for your redness and flushing, you have a couple of good treatment options at your disposal. Recent studies suggest that topical application of 4 percent *nicotinamide* (nonprescription Nicomide-T) may help lessen redness and flushing. In fact, some dermatologists are using topical nicotinamide to alleviate the redness that occurs after laser treatments and with certain medications, including the very strong antiacne drug Accutane.

IPL—the same wonderful in-office treatment that works so well for fading age spots—can help reduce redness and flushing by targeting blood vessels at the surface of the skin. Just as for age spots, your doctor may recommend a series of treatments spaced 2 to 4 weeks apart.

If you decide to go the IPL route, you will be light-years ahead (pardon the pun!) if you ask your doctor to administer multiple pulses over the same area. The treated skin will be left a deep red to almost purplish hue. Please don't be alarmed by this! It's a sign that the blood vessels have thoroughly reacted with the light source. Within a couple of days, the discoloration will disappear—and redness and flushing will be a thing of the past.

IPL is terrific for the face and chest. I love the way it works; to borrow a line I read in *Prevention* magazine, it acts like Windex for the skin. I prefer IPL to the V-beam laser, since the V-beam is vessel-specific whereas the IPL can clear up an entire anatomic area.

Redness Caused by Irritation

If your redness is a sign of irritated skin, you need to do two things: First, treat the irritation; and second, figure out what caused it.

For an at-home treatment, my suggestion is to apply a zinc-based sunscreen. You need to find a very good one, with micronized zinc oxide that goes on thin and isn't sticky. It will help calm your skin and lessen redness. As a bonus, the sunscreen will moisturize your skin and, of course, help protect from sun damage—and more spots and freckles.

Some newer skin lotions, like Eucerin Redness Relief (which contains a licorice derivative), can help reduce redness. So can a hydrocortisone cream in over-the-counter strength.

To determine what's behind the irritation and redness, I'd begin by reexamining the ingredient lists on your skin-care products—keeping a watchful eye for those Poison Ivy ingredients we discussed in Week #2. But identifying the culprit sometimes requires more Sherlock Holmesian methods of observation. Perhaps one of the following two scenarios will ring a bell with you.

REDNESS SCENARIO #1: STRESS

Have you been under a lot of pressure lately, perhaps more so than usual? *Seborrheic dermatitis* is a common response to stress. It causes red, dry, scaly patches on the skin—often in hair-bearing areas, like the eyebrows and hairline, as well as along the sides of the nose and in the creases that run from the nose to the corners of the mouth (the nasolabial folds).

Seborrheic dermatitis responds very well to topical hydrocortisone. I suggest applying a 1 percent hydrocortisone cream twice a day for 1 week, then once a day (at bedtime, if you prefer) for another week. Your skin should heal just fine.

REDNESS SCENARIO #2: ALLERGIC REACTION

Have you recently started wearing a new necklace around your neck or a new fragrance behind your ears? Have you switched shampoos or conditioners? Are you taking a new medication or supplement? If your answer to any of these questions is yes, then your redness may be a sign of an allergic reaction. Here's a rundown of the most common culprits.

Nickel: About 10 percent of the population is allergic to nickel. A lot of women know that they get rashes when they wear nongold jewelry, but they don't realize that even 14-karat gold can leach out nickel.

A company called Allerderm Laboratories offers a kit to test any object for nickel. You can order the Allertest Ni kit by calling (800) 365-6868 or going online to www.allerderm.com. Following the instructions in the kit, you moisten a cotton-tipped applicator with two types of solution, then rub the solution onto the object in question. If the applicator changes color, the object contains nickel.

In the meantime, don't go to bed wearing Grandma's beautiful old necklace until you've had a chance to test it. You could wake up with a red face.

Fragrance: Most of us assume that a fragrance must be artificial to cause irritation and redness. But even botanicals can be problematic for people who are allergic to them. In other words, any product with a strong scent—whether the source of the scent is natural or artificial—could cause a skin reaction. What to do? Eliminate the potential offender from your regimen and apply a 1 percent hydrocortisone cream to the affected area until the redness goes away.

Shampoos and conditioners: Many shampoos and conditioners, among other hair-care products, contain common skin irritants. Especially if you've changed products recently, check the ingredient lists for lanolin, sodium lauryl sulfate, and shea butter—our Poison Ivy ingredients from Week #2. All of them can cause irritation and redness, not to mention acne. (I'll say more about shopping for hair-care products in Week #5.)

Skin-care products: Has redness been a problem for you only since you began your new skin-care regimen? If so, let's try to identify and eliminate any known irritants or at least reduce your exposure to them.

As I've mentioned before, retinol can leave skin red and flaky. Lately I've been seeing this ingredient in all kinds of surprising places, including sunscreens. Glycolic acid—particularly a physician-strength formulation—can cause irritation and redness, sometimes a day or so after use.

Once you've isolated the product that seems to bothering your skin, eliminate it from your regimen for 3 days and nights. If the redness clears, you've found the culprit. This doesn't mean you should give up on the product, especially if you're happy with the results otherwise. You just need to use it less often or switch to a weaker formulation.

Medications and herbal/nutritional supplements: Sometimes a new medicine or supplement can trigger a skin reaction. For example, the herb St. John's wort can make you more sensitive to the sun, while niacin can give you a sudden flush. Read the labels on any herbal or nutritional supplements that you may be taking to see if there are possible skin-related side effects.

Likewise, antibiotics and diuretics (water pills) can increase sun sensitivity, as can hydroquinone and Retin-A. Every once in a while, I hear reports of oral contraceptives causing redness and flushing; some women even break out in acne from it. Since this sort of reaction tends to be hereditary, you might ask your mom whether she had any problems with her skin while she was pregnant.

If you still can't pinpoint what's irritating your skin, you might want to talk with your dermatologist about a patch test for skin allergies. The test includes the 24 substances that most commonly trigger allergic reactions. But each of these 24 things has ties to about 10 other things. So basically, your doctor is testing about 200 possible allergens to determine which might be adversely affecting you.

CAMP ACTIVITY #4
WHAT'S CAUSING YOUR DARK CIRCLES?

No woman wants to see dark undereye circles when she looks in the mirror. If you have them, this camp activity is especially for you. We're going to figure out what's causing your circles, so we can identify an effective strategy for getting rid of them.

Standing before a mirror, gently press under your eyes with your fingertips. Hold for 30 seconds, keeping the pressure constant and even. Now remove your fingers and see what happens.

If you don't see any change in the circles when you stop pressing, it means that they are made totally of pigment. You can treat them much as you would treat an age spot, with a hydroquinone fade preparation.

If the circles seem to disappear, only to reappear within moments, they are caused by increased vascular permeability—that is, the leaking of blood from the veins that run beneath the eyes and between the eyes and nose. A new patented ingredient called Eyeliss not only reduces vascular permeability in very thin-skinned areas, such as around the eyes, it also increases the contraction of lymphatic vessels to draw away the fluid that collects under the eyes. So circles aren't as visible, and they aren't as heavy, either. The three active substances in Eyeliss help restore elasticity and firmness to the skin, too.

Eyeliss already has been incorporated into several skin-care products. Perhaps you've seen those attention-grabbing ads with the thick black lines drawn under a young model's eyes. I recently started using an Eyeliss product myself; it really does work. In fact, it lessened my undereye circles so dramatically that my daughter Gina thought I'd had eye surgery.

Another effective ingredient for treating purplish, vascular undereye circles is topical vitamin K. Products that contain the vitamin tend to be marketed as such, so look for a mention of vitamin K in either the product name or action name. (For a refresher course on action names, please refer to Week #2.)

Suppose you get a mixed result from the finger-pressure test: Your circles don't completely go away when you stop pressing, but they are less noticeable when you lift your fingers. You need to address both issues—excess pigment and increased vascular permeability—by using a hydroquinone preparation and an Eyeliss product simulatenously.

CAMP ACTIVITY #5
MENDING BROKEN BLOOD VESSELS

Broken capillaries and blood vessels can have any number of causes. Sometimes they reflect a high estrogen state, which is why both pregnancy and oral contraceptive use can be contributing factors. So too, can excessive alcohol consumption—or any other behavior that could result in liver damage, since estrogen normally is broken down in the liver. (People with unhealthy livers look like they have too much estrogen. Men with liver disease can even develop enlarged breasts and broken vessels.)

Sometimes broken blood vessels are more hereditary in nature. Many a redheaded patient has complained to me that as soon as she turned 40, her face erupted in broken or enlarged blood vessels. Redheads can inherit a tendency toward fair, freckling skin, which makes them very sensitive to the sun and therefore more likely to burn, freckle, and develop broken vessels over time. I've noticed, too, how many women come into my office for removal of broken vessels they claim are carbon copies of those that appeared on their moms' faces at about the same age.

Unfortunately, some broken blood vessels can be somewhat self-inflicted. A strong glycolic acid product can bring them on, as can Renova and Retin-A. Be sure to read the cautions on skin-care products such as these, and take care not to apply them in areas where you already have broken vessels. Usually, if you discontinue treatment for a while, minor broken vessels will clear up by themselves.

Some women with broken blood vessels see improvement once they begin using topical vitamin K or a prescription rosacea medication. If your complaint is just a few isolated broken vessels, such as on the sides of your nose, the V-beam laser is the gold standard.

When it first came out, the V-beam was touted for producing less immediate posttreatment disfigurement and therefore requiring less significant recovery time. Since then, we've learned that to effectively eliminate unwanted broken blood vessels with a laser, we need to induce *purpura*, or a dark purpling of the vessel. Otherwise, the vessel won't completely disappear. Though the dark purple color is temporary, it is almost impossible to cover up, even with the heaviest concealers and scar makeup. And since most broken vessels appear smack-dab in the center of the face—usually as a network of red spidery veins on the sides of the nose—the patient will have significant downtime (about a week to 10 days for a facial procedure).

The cost of a V-beam treatment session runs between $250 and $400. One session may be enough, though sometimes treatment needs to be repeated.

. . . .

SCARY CAMP STORY:
THE PILL AND BROKEN VESSELS

A couple of years ago, a woman in her late twenties came to my office, seeking help with some bothersome broken blood vessels. They were concentrated around her nose, though a few had surfaced on her chest. She was rather confused by the opinions of the dermatologists she already had seen, each of whom had recommended a different laser as the best "cure."

In cases like this, I like to gather more history from the patient, so I can determine the cause of the problem and recommend the best treatment. This woman told me that she had been on oral contraceptives continuously for 6 years. When I asked her if she thought the broken blood vessels were getting worse, she said yes. They had a certain shape that we doctors call spiders, with a very red center and fine leglike projections radiating outward.

I explained to her that spider-type broken vessels often occur in the presence of a high-estrogen state, such as pregnancy or oral contraceptive use. In my opinion, she most definitely had developed the spiders as a side effect of the birth control pills. I advised her to switch her method of contraception, as it would be the best way to treat the broken vessels.

When this patient returned for her follow-up, she told me that she had taken my advice—although reluctantly. Three months later, her spiders were barely visible; 6 months later, there was no trace of them.

CAMP LESSON
SOME NEW THOUGHTS ABOUT SUN PROTECTION

I'm always alarmed when I see extensive freckling on the back of a patient who's still in her twenties. Those large freckles reveal overexposure to the sun's ultraviolet rays at an early age—and they could foretell a higher risk of skin cancer later in life. Practicing as I do in Miami Beach, with its large population of boaters and sunbathers, I am saddened by this tendency toward solar excess.

And yet . . . even though I'm a dermatologist, I must admit that lightly tanned skin looks much healthier to me than milky whiteness. When I see someone who's very pale, my gut reaction is to wonder whether the person is sick. My reaction is driven in part by our sun-worshipping culture. But it also arises from my medical knowledge that sun exposure can be therapeutic, particularly for seriously ill patients. Also, research proves that sun deprivation can lead to depression.

A growing body of evidence suggests that we should not be shielding ourselves from the sun at all times. Vincent DeLeo, MD, a well-respected dermatologist at Columbia University, speculates that because of rampant widespread sunscreen use, many of us are not producing enough natural vitamin D to ensure healthy bones. Further, Dr. DeLeo cautions, we don't have good established guidelines for vitamin D replacement.

His observations have persuaded some people to at least consider spending time outdoors without any sunscreen.

What's my opinion? Certainly, more than 95 percent of skin cancers come from excessive sun exposure—and the damage done by the sun is more than just unhealthy. It is unsightly. If you doubt me, just compare the skin on sun-exposed parts of your body (like your face, chest, and shoulders) with the skin on unexposed parts. By the time you reach your fifties, your buttocks probably look decades younger than the rest of your skin—unless you've done a great deal of nude sunbathing or you've been very diligent about safeguarding your skin from the sun.

So my advice is this: Enjoy the sun, but protect your skin. And the most effective measure for preventing age spots and wrinkles, as well as skin cancer, is to wear sunscreen on any exposed areas. The trick is to find a sunscreen that truly blocks the sun.

I know what you're thinking: How could we get more specific than an SPF? But these ratings have a serious flaw: They are determined by a laboratory test that measures protection against UVB rays. Most dermatologists agree that the rise in melanomas—not to mention skin discolorations and skin aging—is the result of exposure to UVA rays, the most harmful in the ultraviolet spectrum.

Unfortunately, we don't have a good, reliable test for UVA protection just yet. So you can go out and buy a product with an SPF 15 or even 70 and still know next to nothing about whether the product effectively blocks the most dangerous of the sun's rays.

How do I protect my skin from the sun? By following the

Tanning without the Sun

The self-tanners currently on the market have come a long way since the products of my teens and twenties. They contain dihydroxyacetone, an ingredient that combines with the dead skin cells of the stratum corneum, giving the skin a harmless but (I think) attractive hue. Usually just a single application is enough.

Many of my younger patients who otherwise see no need for a skin-care regimen are crazy for a Jergens product called Natural Glow, a moisturizer that contains a very small amount of dihydroxyacetone. Many moms who worry about their teenagers tanning now and paying later might consider Natural Glow as an alternative. It's available in both face and body lotions.

If you're wondering whether you should try a self-tanner, slip on a favorite skirt or pair of shorts. How do your legs look? Would they look better with a touch of color? Some of my patients have said that using self-tanner makes their legs appear slimmer and shapelier, just as wearing 2-inch heels can—but the tanner is much more comfortable. It works for me, and it just might work for you!

dermatologists' party line on the most basic protocol. When I am going to the beach or a picnic or spending the day on a boat, I slather my skin with a waterproof sunscreen that will shield my skin from UVA rays. I know this because the sunscreen contains zinc oxide (my personal favorite), titanium dioxide, or Parsol (a chemical filter that blocks UVA).

With sunscreens, as with all skin-care products, reading labels is critical. It's a bit easier here, though, since sunscreens are classified as over-the-counter drugs and therefore must follow a strict labeling format established by the FDA. The sun-protection agent—the active ingredient—always appears first in the ingredient list.

For anyone who is extrasensitive to the sun or spends most of her days outdoors, I recommend a terrific product called Rit Sun Guard Laundry Treatment UV Protectant. Add it to a load of laundry, and it makes clothes sun protective (roughly the equivalent of SFP 30) for the next 20 washes.

Week #4 Review

- *We live in a wrinkle-obsessed world. For many of us, though, improving our skin tone can make more of a difference in our appearance than erasing those tiny lip lines.*
- *Fine-tune your skin-care regimen to target any age spots, discolorations, redness, dark circles, or broken blood vessels.*
- *Sometimes rosacea isn't rosacea—it's the wasabi crackers.*
- *Don't hide from the sun! Finding a good sunscreen and using it every day is a great solution to enjoying the outdoors while protecting your skin.*
- *Don't be intimidated by your dermatologist, or by any doctor. Ask all the questions you need to, and get all the answers you expect.*
- *Are you getting 30 extra minutes of sleep? Are you seeing a difference?*
- *Do those facial exercises!*

Week #5

Your Hair and Makeup
This week's agenda:
Getting your whole act together

For me, hair and makeup—and what I do or don't do with them—has as much impact on my appearance as getting enough sleep, doing my facial exercises, and using the right skin-care products. Since I think this is true for most of us, I want to be sure that you give sufficient time and attention to this week's agenda.

Let's start by taking another look at your Orientation photos—only this time, focusing on your hair. And by "hair," I mean *all* of it—including your eyebrows, any peach fuzz (or worse) above your lip, and any strays on your chin.

Are your eyebrows well groomed? Sometimes a simple shaping (by plucking the stray hairs with tweezers, as I often do, or by professional waxing) can lift and open your eyes dramatically. As some very good "eyebrow professionals" have told me, they offer a great quick and inexpensive alternative to an eye job!

As for those unwanted facial hairs, we'll take care of those, too. There's a great new topical preparation called Vaniqa that can actually stop facial hair from growing. I'll tell you more about it later.

Your hairstyle—both the cut and the color—serves as a frame for your face, much like a frame for a painting. I've been known to purchase a $20 print at a street stand while on vacation, put it in a beautiful frame—and transform it into a piece of art that I am proud to display in my home. Now is the time to ask whether your hair is the best frame for your face. Is it doing justice to your features?

Just as we get into ruts with our skin-care regimens and continue using products that don't work for us anymore, we can become attached to a certain hairstyle that just doesn't enhance our best features. Old habits die hard! Then, too, we may feel that we simply don't have the time, energy, or budget to "reinvent" our hair.

But here you are at Beauty Camp—and it's Week #5 already! By now you definitely should be seeing a payoff from updating your skin-care regimen. Your skin is healthier, smoother, and free from distracting spots and discolorations. It shouldn't be overshadowed by an outdated hairdo.

I know what you may be thinking: *She isn't a hairstylist or a makeup artist.* But I do care about my appearance. My hair is an important aspect of looking my best. I work to keep it healthy and attractive and styled in a way that flatters my face. When did you last change your hairstyle? When were you last tempted?

CAMP ACTIVITY #1

THE BEST 'DO FOR YOU

Most of us have gone through at least a few hairstyles in our lives, even if not in the recent past. It might be helpful to review them now. Find a few older photos of yourself in which you're wearing your hair differently than you do now. They might reveal whether you look better with one length or another. If you've kept your hair long and straight for years, try to find a photo in which it's pulled back in a ponytail or pinned away from your face.

Gather these photos and take them into the bathroom. Stand in front of the mirror and really study your hair. Does it complement your face as well as it could? Among the factors that you should consider:

1. Is your hair the right length for you?
2. Are you happy with the color?
3. Is your hair healthy and shiny?
4. Do you notice any thinning?

Looking at your old photos, do you see a cut or color that's more flattering than your current style? Even if you're certain that you already have the perfect hair for your age and face, I urge you to be open to change. What do you have to lose?

Another good idea is to get a second opinion—especially if you have any sentimental attachment to your current hairstyle. I love asking my kids about my hair. They've known me through countless changes, and they have a good sense of what's most flattering to my face. They don't pull any punches, either. But they've yet to steer me wrong. While I don't wear much makeup, sometimes my daughters offer suggestions about that, too.

I wonder if you have somebody like that in your life—somebody whom you can count on to be honest and helpful. All of us could use another pair of eyes and a fresh perspective. Often people are hesitant to express an opinion, especially on matters of appearance—unless someone asks for their input. So why not ask?

I definitely would make a point of seeking the opinion of someone younger—perhaps a son or daughter, a niece or nephew, a neighbor, the intern in your office. This person should have a keen eye and a good sense of style (though not because I want you to start wearing the latest teenage fashions). Your purpose here is to fish for options and possibilities that you may not have considered otherwise.

That Magic Length

According to the conventional wisdom, women look better with shorter hair as they get older. This may be true, to a degree. For example, if you wore your hair straight down your back all through your twenties and thirties, it might be a good idea to trim a few inches once you're in your forties.

Women in their forties to sixties tend to look best with hair that falls somewhere between the chin and shoulders, so it sweeps under the jawline. This can take years off your face. If you're hesitant to try it, you might start by asking your stylist to cut just a few wisps of hair right around your face so that they hug your chin. See what a difference this can make!

Very few women can pull off supershort hair. It requires excellent facial symmetry and soft features—or one knockout feature, like almond-shaped sky-blue eyes. But on older women especially, short hair can look matronly and severe. It also may draw attention to a sagging jawline or crinkled neck.

If your hair seems too short, you may want to try growing it a bit—say, to chin length. I know this isn't easy; your hair will probably go through a few awkward stages. But a good stylist can help with transitional cuts that will keep your hair looking neat. If you're worried that growing out your hair won't be worth the effort, you might visit a wig shop and ask to try on a few longer styles to get a better sense of how you'll look. Also, some salons advertise computer software that lets you sample styles on a digital image of your face.

If your hair is already long, try tucking it under to see if wearing it shorter would lift your face. Is shoulder length better? How about chin length? If you have jowls or even just a little sagging at the jawline, cutting your hair so that it falls between your chin and shoulders could help soften or camouflage this Uninvited Element (UE).

In fact, think for a moment about all the ways in which a new hairstyle could minimize or balance something about your face that you aren't crazy about. In my case, pulling my hair away from my face reveals my very small temples. So I always have a cut that camouflages what I view as a flaw in the shape of my face.

Fashion and lifestyle magazines are filled with photos of actresses and models who use their hair to downplay or enhance certain facial features. For example, celebrity women over age 50 seem to prefer long bangs, almost in their eyes. It's a good trick for concealing a furrowed brow and drawing attention away from crow's-feet. It also seems to erase years from the

Consult a Pro

A good stylist and a good colorist are essential for great-looking hair. (If you can find one person who excels at both skills, consider yourself blessed!) Now is an opportune time to think about whether you're happy with the services you've been getting. Searching for someone new isn't a betrayal.

Ask your fellow Beauty Campers or your friends or co-workers who does their hair. Exchange information about local salons and the services they provide. In my experience, salons can vary greatly in the time and attention they give to customers and in the quality of the hair-care products they use.

If you see someone with magnificent hair, ask who her stylist or colorist is and which salon she goes to. Doing this isn't so hard; just be on the lookout at the office and supermarket, even in the line for the ATM. Don't worry if the woman is a total stranger. More than likely, she'll be flattered by your compliment—and happy to refer a new client to her stylist or colorist.

I found my colorist exactly this way, through a patient who had come into my office for a Botox treatment. She

face, as I discovered a few months ago, when I took the scissors to my own hair and created bangs. Other older women frame their faces with volumes of tousled hair—possibly to hide cosmetic surgery scars or flatter a face that's gotten heavier.

was in a big hurry, she said, and late for an appointment at a salon. I must confess that, as soon as she mentioned her hair, I began to really study it. The color was fabulous. I picked up my mirror (which is very unforgiving under the fluorescent lights of an exam room) and took a good look at my own color.

"Susan," I said, "your hair looks so much healthier than mine! And the color is much more compatible with your skin tone." That's when I switched to a new colorist and never looked back.

It's fine to stick with your current stylist or colorist, of course. Just be sure to tell him that you're coming in for a consultation to discuss changing your hairstyle or color. Try to schedule this appointment for a slower time in the salon, especially if your stylist or colorist tends to be so busy that he barely can catch his breath, much less assess whether your hair is complementing your face.

Once I get into a salon chair, I leave a lot of the decision making to the expert. Give thought to your style and color, but also allow your stylist or colorist a reasonable amount of free rein. At the very least, your hair will grow out if the results aren't what you hoped for.

Younger women take advantage of these styling tricks, too. It's possible to hide a too-full face or wide jaw with a hairstyle that sweeps over it. (Have you ever noticed how Jennifer Aniston's hair always covers the sides of her face?)

In some ways, our hair is even more important than our skin in creating an overall impression. All of us look our best with hair that's the right length and style and in good condition. If yours isn't, then it may be time to make a change—or at least to seriously contemplate one.

Really Good Color

While you're studying the length and style of your hair, take note of the color. Does it look healthy and natural? Or does it remind you of—for want of a better description—a sack of straw?

The rule of thumb about color is that as we get older, we should go slightly darker rather than lighter. This is because the eye can perceive blonde tones as gray. (Did you happen to see the movie *The Hours*? If so, you might recall how actress Julianne Moore's hair went from a beautiful, vibrant red to a cross between platinum blonde and gray, to suggest the passage of time.) If you love your blonde color, consider adding some lowlights—darker tones—the next time you visit your colorist.

This Thin Isn't In

Many patients are surprised when I tell them that a woman's hair usually begins to recede by her early thirties. She also may notice that her hair isn't quite as thick and plentiful as it once was.

There are multiple reasons for these changes, with aging itself bearing just some of the blame. All the stuff that we do to our hair—from traction (pulling it into a ponytail, for example) to coloring (sensitivity to dyes can lead to low-grade inflammation of the scalp)—contributes to the fact that many of us have less of it in our forties than we did in our thirties. So, too, do more traumatic life events like stress and childbirth. (I temporarily lost a lot of hair with the birth of each of my children.)

If you want to thicken your hair, I recommend using Nioxin hair-care products. Nioxin can be a near-miracle product line for regrowing hair. Apparently, word of Nioxin spread after chemotherapy nurses who had been providing it to their patients began recommending it to their friends and neighbors, as well. I must admit that I love it, too!

What about trying minoxidil—or the brand-name product Rogaine—for thinning hair? Two cautions here: First, the manufacturer developed Women's Rogaine (a 2 percent formulation) after some women who had been using the original product (5 percent formulation) began sprouting facial hair. So if you must try it, please use only the lower strength. But here's the real scoop: Once you start treatment, your hair could fall out if you stop.

This is why I recommend trying a Nioxin product first. If you don't get the results you expect within a couple of months, then you might consider Women's Rogaine.

EXTREME CHALLENGE
IS YOUR HAIR REALLY THINNING?

If your hair seems to be thinning more rapidly than normal, you may want to do a couple of tests to see whether your hair loss really is significant.

First, let's count how many hairs you actually lose in a day. To prepare, you'll need to thoroughly clean your comb and brush of all hair. Also, make sure that not a single strand remains in your shower stall, on your bathroom floor, on your pillowcase, or anyplace else that hair tends to cling.

On the morning of the test, wash your hair. Then keep a running tally of the number of hairs that fall out over the course of the day—in your brush and comb, on the bathroom counter and floor, on the shoulders of your sweater, on your pillow, and so on.

The average person loses up to 100 hairs a day. If your count is below that, then you probably don't have a medical condition that could be contributing to your thinning hair. (Incidentally, even men with male pattern baldness don't lose a lot of hairs every day. But when thick hairs fall out, baby-fine strands take their place.)

If your count exceeds 100, you might want to check the potential side effects of any medications you take. I've found that certain heart drugs, blood pressure pills, and other prescription medicines can lead to significant hair loss. You also might ask your doctor about screenings for anemia or thyroid irregularities. (Depending on any other symptoms that you may have, your doctor may screen for lupus, too.)

Suppose your count is under 100, but your hair definitely is thinning. Then do the second test. This one takes just a moment—I promise!

Make a good, straight center part in your hair. Does it seem wider than it did in the past? If so, you are experiencing true hair thinning. You need to at least start treatment with Nioxin.

More often than not, women—and some men—are reassured when they do these tests. For example, some women discover that their only problem is too-long hair, which makes the

50 or so hairs that they lose in a day seem like a lot more. Parts may look wider in women who color their hair darker, but it's only an illusion. A pale scalp always seems more pronounced with dark hair.

CAMP ACTIVITY #2
HAIR-CARE PRODUCTS THAT CAUSE ACNE

If your goal is truly clear—that's right, smooth and spotless—skin, then you really must heed my advice about hair-care products. A number of these products are potentially comedogenic, or acne-causing. Even when you rinse them out of your hair, they leave behind a residue that eventually dries into deposits on your face.

Some of my patients can't believe that their shampoos, conditioners, or styling products may be to blame for their skin problems. In fact, these products can irritate the skin, leading to redness, rashes, and full-blown breakouts. I've seen patients left with stubborn brown spots and stains, the "scars" of doing battle against this kind of skin flare-up.

To see if what you use on your hair may be affecting your skin, let's head back into the bathroom under those bright lights. Study your face in the mirror. Do you notice any redness or tiny bumps? Are they clustered at the periphery of your face? Gently pull your hair away from your face. Does this expose the most troublesome areas? If so, you must change your hair-care products as soon as possible. These tips will help you choose wisely—and heal your skin quickly.

1. Think clearly about shampoo. Look for one that is translucent, never opaque, pearly, or creamy. (Neutrogena Clear, with sodium bureth sulfate, is a good example.) If you are sensitive to fragrance, make sure the shampoo is fragrance free or at least not heavily perfumed.

2. Skip creamy conditioners. These can leave potentially comedogenic molecules on your hair, which will dry and flake onto your forehead and along the sides of your face. The problem is tenfold with creamy leave-in conditioners. As an alternative, I have complete faith in a product called Infusium 23 Leave-In Treatment, which comes with a spout applicator. If you have colored hair, which tends to be dull, you might try a leave-in "shine" or silicone product. I like Frizz-Ease Down-Play Volume Reducer.

If you just can't part with your creamy conditioner because nothing else seems to make your hair look as good, then follow your conditioning treatment by washing your face with a good salicylic acid cleanser. Pay particular attention to the skin around your hairline and neck.

3. Choose mousse over gel. Many people find that the prolonged use of hair gels can enlarge or stretch their pores because the products are so thick. Hair sprays won't hurt your skin, but they do tend to dry out hair.

4. Invest in a good-quality plastic shower cap. Hopefully, you picked up a shower cap way back at Orientation. If not, now is the time to get one. A shower cap will protect your hair from the dampness and humidity of your daily shower. Anytime your hair gets damp or wet and then dries out, it loses some of its essential oils and natural conditioning. We want your hair to look healthy and hydrated, not dry and dull.

Along the same line, if you live in a rainy climate, you might

What about the Hair . . . There?

Take a very close look at your upper lip and chin. As we women age, we can sprout new growth in these areas.

You probably are familiar with the most common methods of removing unwanted facial hair. To recap, they include bleaching (downside: the hair is blonde, but it still is there), waxing (can cause rashes and breakouts), depilatory creams such as Nair (require more frequent use than waxing), and shaving (5 o'clock shadow). Of these, bleaching and waxing are equally good bets in terms of effectiveness and safety.

A prescription topical preparation called Vaniqa works well for preventing the growth of unwanted facial hair. The instructions for Vaniqa suggest that women shave their faces before applying the product. In my experience, it works just fine without that step.

Among the available in-office options for facial hair removal is the Alexandrite laser. It's extremely safe, but since it works by destroying pigment, it's effective only if you have dark hair and light skin.

Another increasingly popular method of hair removal is intense pulsed light (IPL), which we discussed in Week #4. Although it doesn't produce the dramatic results of the Alexandrite laser, IPL can get rid of lighter-colored facial hairs, which the Alexandrite cannot. IPL treatments are less expensive, too.

want to invest in a plastic rain hat—the kind that you can fold up and keep in your purse or coat pocket. Then, if you get caught in the rain without an umbrella, you won't need to wash your hair when you get home.

5. Shampoo less frequently. The more you wash your hair, the drier it becomes. The drier it becomes, the more moisturizing it requires—and the more potentially problematic hair-care products it absorbs.

It's true that the best products help moisturize hair. In my experience, though, the best way to "moisturize" is to simply cut back on shampooing. Then your hair's essential oils can do their job.

Most women should be able to get by with shampooing just once or twice a week. Those who restyle their hair frequently might shampoo 1 day a week and simply rinse with water on other days.

If you must wash your hair several times a week, try shampooing just once rather than following the "lather-rinse-repeat" instruction that seems to be standard on product labels. What if you have oily hair that requires more frequent cleansing? Here's an idea: Wash with a clear shampoo and skip the conditioner. Generally, oily hair doesn't need conditioning and isn't likely to dry out from overwashing.

CAMP ACTIVITY #3
REVAMPING YOUR MAKEUP

Makeup, when done well, can do wonders for a woman's appearance and self-confidence. Just ask any of my patients who've seen me in my office one day and live on *Good Morning America* the next. The show's stylists are amazing!

A friend of mine who happens to know Bobbi Brown, a makeup artist and *Prevention* magazine columnist, still talks about the time that Bobbi appeared on her doorstep to administer some much-needed "beauty therapy." My friend had been going through a difficult divorce, and her husband had moved out just the day before. Makeup kit in hand, Bobbi redid my friend's face. Thinking back on that experience, she says that Bobbi did more for her than any psychotherapist could have.

What you do with your makeup can run the gamut from subtly correcting "flaws" to dramatically enhancing facial features. As with your hair, the big question about your makeup is this: When was the last time you changed it? If you've been using the same products for years, they may actually be dating you. You want people to notice your clear, smooth skin—not that gaudy shade of eye shadow or lipstick.

For some fresh ideas, browse through the photos in your favorite beauty and lifestyle magazines. After all, you probably wouldn't think of renovating your kitchen without first studying an armload of shelter magazines. Changing your makeup calls for the same consideration. As you thumb through magazines, do you see any looks you like?

Also pay attention to the makeup of the women around you—your sisters, friends, co-workers, and, of course, fellow Beauty Campers. Though you don't want to duplicate their looks, you may learn something from their product choices and techniques.

Getting a Professional Makeover

All of us have seen those women patiently perched on the stools at department-store cosmetics counters and beauty boutiques, where makeup artists create a "new look" just for them. Such a personal consultation isn't a bad idea, especially if you've been using the same makeup for a while. Even if you don't like the end result, I'll bet one or two recommendations will appeal to you. There's something to be learned from every experience!

If you can't bear the notion of getting a makeover in a public setting, you might be able to find a makeup artist who makes house calls. If you're among a group of Beauty Campers, perhaps he or she would be willing to attend a meeting.

Another option is to rent an instructional video or DVD. In fact, several cosmetic lines offer free videos if you buy their products. Model Lauren Hutton, who is in her sixties and looks incredible, has created a cosmetic line for older skin. Her products come with a very good video, in which she demonstrates how to use makeup creatively and intelligently.

Your Foundation

Now that your skin is becoming smooth and healthy, with fewer spots and stains to conceal, why cover it with foundation? My advice is to skip the foundation and face powder altogether, or use as little as possible. With foundation, you run the risk of accentuating pores and fine lines. On my face, I prefer a lightly tinted moisturizer with sunscreen, plus a mineral powder in areas that tend to be a little blotchy, like my nose. The powder helps brighten skin and minimize any remaining imperfections.

Your Eye Makeup

Let's start with your eyebrows. They can be shaped in a way that nicely frames your eyes or distracts from any crow's-feet or undereye puffiness by drawing attention upward. See what happens if you emphasize them a bit. After grooming them, you might apply either eyebrow mascara (I love the one from Victoria's Secret, which comes in clear or several shades of brown) or a light shade of eye shadow, brushing it into your brows. This highlights the arch of the brow ever so slightly, enhancing the facial aesthetic.

If your eyes are small, a light beige or putty-colored shadow can make them appear larger, especially if you apply it at the corners of the eyes and right beneath the brows. You might also try using shadow as eyeliner—line one lid with powder and another with liquid liner. Which works best for enhancing your eye color and contour?

Most women seem to prefer eye pencils for lining, but I would encourage you to experiment with shadows and liquid liners, too. You can find a multitude of products at a variety of price points; my guess is that many of them come from the same manufacturer but carry different labels. So go to the drugstore and buy one or two.

As for color, I'd steer clear of black, at least to start. It's a little too severe for most eyes. If you're trying eyeliner for the first time, go with a soft brown or my personal favorite—violet.

You'll be amazed at how violet hues complement your eye color, especially if you have green or hazel eyes.

There's a common misconception that eyeliner makes eyes seem smaller. It all depends how you apply it. My friend Lillian taught me a trick for using liner that creates the illusion of size and fullness.

Lillian is a former actress who gave up the silver screen when she married and moved to Florida. While in Hollywood, she'd been great pals with the Gabor sisters, Zsa Zsa and Eva, who showed Lillian how they made their rather small eyes appear magnificently large and exotic on camera. Their secret? When applying liner to their top and bottom eyelids, they never let the lines meet at the outside corner of the eye. When they wore liner only on the top lid, they extended the line just a bit beyond the eye, with a slight upward turn at the outer corner.

Try both of these techniques to see which you like best. I've tried them, too, and they definitely work. Once you choose your favorite technique, see what happens when you make each line slightly thicker. If you like the look, you may want to switch to liquid eyeliner, just because it will stay in place for most of the day—unlike eye pencils, which are notorious for smudging and fading.

Thanks to my friend Lillian for the marvelous tips—and to the Gabor sisters for sharing their knowledge with Lillian.

Lip Color and Shine

Before any woman rushes into injections to enhance her lip size, she owes it to herself to see what some lip liner and color can do. Gather up all the lipsticks you have—from your bathroom, vanity, and purse. You may be able to achieve the fullness you're looking for by wearing several layers of color at once. Give it a try!

Since my mouth is wide, I prefer to wear softer shades of lipstick and gloss, like pinks and beiges. Remember that certain lip colors can cause teeth to appear discolored. To keep mine looking white, I use a whitening product called Rembrandt Whitening Wand. I picked it up at a drugstore on Christmas Eve several years ago, when I was in a last-minute rush for stocking stuffers. It fits easily into my purse; I've carried it with me ever since.

Cosmetics, Etc.

As for the rest of your makeup, I suggest keeping it simple. Just think about how you react when you see a woman who's gone even a tad overboard with the cosmetics. Makeup should enhance your appearance, not detract from it. Halloween comes once a year. Don't be caught in costume!

Once you've put on your "face" for the day, remember that the best finishing touch is a smile. Studies confirm that women who are frequent smilers are more sexually attractive to men. Isn't that funny? All the stuff we worry about—laugh lines, crow's-feet, spots and stains—may not matter as much as we think. Perhaps the easiest way to improve our appearance is to show those pearly whites.

CAMP ACTIVITY #4
SHARING YOUR LOOT

Back in Week #2 of Beauty Camp, I asked you to collect all of your cosmetics, as well as your hair- and skin-care products, into one big box. If you skipped the cosmetics at the time, go grab them now. Remember to search through your bathroom cabinet and drawers, vanity, purse, and briefcase. We want to see every single item that you've purchased to color, conceal, and enhance, whether or not you've actually used them all.

Just as we did with your skin-care products, let's organize everything into three piles: Not-Sures, Discards, and Essentials. You probably don't need all 10 of those lipsticks that are exactly the same shade. (Aren't they too dark anyway?) You can't remember when you bought that bottle of foundation. And the bright blue eye shadow . . . what were you thinking?

Once you have your three piles, let's concentrate on the Not-Sures for a moment. You might want to pick through this pile with a friend or two or with your fellow Beauty Campers. Ask for their opinions on the various products and colors. They can help you whittle down the pile until you're left with mostly Discards and Essentials.

Now, about that Discard pile . . . these are the cosmetics that aren't the right color, don't go on smoothly—for one reason or another—haven't worked for you. You could hand them over to someone else, perhaps in exchange for an item from her Discards. Or you could donate them to your household Halloween costume box. (I just did that with a peculiar red lipstick that I found in my drawer.)

Yes, It's Safe to Share

I can guess what you might be thinking: *A dermatologist is telling me to share makeup?!* I sure am! My daughters and I use each other's cosmetics and skin-care products all the time, and we have never run into trouble. True, it's among family. But I can support my personal experience with hard scientific evidence.

About 10 years ago, when I first started doing a weekly spot on a morning television show in Miami, we decided to have a bunch of women in the newsroom bring in makeup they hadn't used for a while. Was it still safe? Or was it rife with germs and other microbes?

Generally, we dermatologists recommend that once a cosmetic has been opened, it should be thrown away after 2 years because the preservatives won't be effective much longer than that. The funny thing is, when we tested some really old mascaras—even tubes that had been opened 4 years earlier and used infrequently—we didn't find any bacteria or other unwanted microbes when we cultured the products in the laboratory.

So what is the risk of sharing makeup with someone else? In my 25 years of dermatologic practice, I have never had a patient come to me with an infection or sore caused by a "communal" cosmetic or cosmetic tester. Sharing shouldn't be a problem, as long as you proceed with a modicum of common sense. For example, you definitely don't want to use makeup from someone with a contagious illness such as a cold or the flu. The same rule applies to sharing with someone with inflamed or pustular acne or eczema, since her skin may harbor a bacterial overgrowth that could contaminate any cosmetic she handles.

If you still feel squeamish about sharing, you can take steps to protect yourself. Use new disposable foam applicators when testing foundations and lipsticks. Bring your own clean makeup brushes for eye shadows and blushes. Sharpen an eye pencil before using it, or dip the tip in rubbing alcohol. (This works for lipstick, too.)

Go Ahead—Have Fun!

I truly believe that sharing and sampling cosmetics is the best way to get a sense of what's on the market and what might work for you. To be sure, the choices are overwhelming. You easily could spend a small fortune in your quest for just the right eye shadow or lipstick. (Perhaps you already have.) Or you could find your favorite new shade with help from a fellow Beauty Camper and her makeup kit (which is how I happily discovered Victoria's Secret Pure Reflection Ultra-Shine Lipstick Fizz #165).

Of all the camp activities so far, this is the one that I sincerely hope you'll consider doing as a group—if not with other Beauty Campers, then with a circle of close friends. It's meant to be relaxed and fun. You might set the mood with wine spritzers and some smooth jazz. Ask everyone to bring their own boxes of cosmetics so you can go through them together. Tell each other which items you can't live without and which you'd forgotten you'd bought. Test them, trade them, and talk about them. The more products, the better!

Before the meeting, several of you could chip in to purchase a few expensive cosmetics that you're eager to try. Or you could canvass local department stores in search of samples. (While you're out and about, be sure to pick up a pack of those disposable foam applicators for sharing products.)

Depending on the age range in your group, you might want

to check out the growing number of cosmetics specifically for middle-age or "mature" skin. For example, Giorgio Armani has a new makeup line made with a fine silicone base that's excellent for mature skin. Revlon, Olay, and Neutrogena also are marketing cosmetics for older women; they're available in most drugstores and supermarkets.

Self-tanners are fantastic for sharing—you'll know how well you like them after just an application or two. Most drugstores and supermarkets carry quite a few reliable brands, such as Neutrogena and Coppertone. Department-store brands tend to be pricier—but some women swear by Clarins and Lancôme.

In the end, some women will leave your group session with thickly lined eyelids, others with just a hint of color on their eyebrows and lots of mascara and still others with the knowledge that their lips really are pretty in pink. The take-home lesson for everyone is this: After you've put so much effort into improving your skin, it's fun—and potentially very rewarding—to see what you can gain from a few tweaks (as my editor would say.) to your makeup routine.

Week #5 Review

- *Find a hairstyle that frames and flatters your face.*
- *Don't go too short or too blonde.*
- *Study the ingredient labels on your hair-care products!*
- *Wash your hair less often—say, once or twice a week at most.*
- *Experiment with your makeup—is it time for a change?*
- *Feel free to share cosmetics as long as you follow a few commonsense safety guidelines.*

- *Keep up treatments for age spots and other skin discolorations.*
- *Take a short break from any glycolic acid or retinol products that may be causing irritation and redness.*
- *Keep those pillowcases clean!*
- *How are you doing on the 30 extra minutes of sleep a night?*
- *Smile!*

Week #6

Reevaluating Your Face

This week's agenda: Assessing and fine-tuning
your skin-care regimen

I always feel a little sad as we get closer to the end of Beauty
Camp. I feel a little nervous, too. How well has my advice
worked for you? By now you should be seeing significant
improvement in your skin. Most campers report fewer fine
lines, smaller pores, and less redness, along with fading of any
age spots or other discolorations.

It's time to ask yourself whether you're satisfied with the
skin-care regimen you're following and the progress you're seeing. Perhaps you've created the absolute best regimen for you,
and you don't need to change a single thing. What more could
you possibly want to know or do? If this describes you, then I
have just one word to say: *Bravo!*

On the other hand, perhaps you're seeing less dramatic
results, even though you've been following my instructions to
the letter. You came to Beauty Camp with expectations that
haven't been met. You might be saying, "Wait—that's it?!"
If this sounds more like you, then this week's activities are

especially for you. We'll be honing in on certain Uninvited Elements (UEs) that may require special attention. We'll also explore a number of tricks and techniques to ramp up your skin-care regimen.

Not all Beauty Campers will want to follow through on these measures right away. You might not be ready for neuro-peptides, Retin-A, or a series of at-home peels. But the time may come when you are. So hang on to this book. It could come in handy down the road.

I have a motto for this week of Beauty Camp: Ramp up—but don't give up.

CAMP ACTIVITY #1
THE DAY OF RECKONING

It's time to get out that camera once again. You are going to take new photos of your face. But first, refer back to the ones that you had taken 5 weeks ago, at the very beginning of Beauty Camp. Try to duplicate the lighting, angles, and facial expressions from the original shoot. We want the photos to be as comparable as possible.

Don't cheat and try to "doctor" your appearance to look better (or worse) than you did 5 weeks ago. If you've created a good skin-care regimen and been diligent about following it, you should see noticeable and possibly dramatic improvements in your skin.

Study your before-and-after photos. If you need help comparing them, share them with a family member or friend, or with your fellow Beauty Campers. Then, under "Improvements" in the space below, write down any changes that you see—better skin tone and health, fewer fine lines and grooves, less redness and discoloration. Be generous and give yourself credit. Did you wrestle a few age spots into submission? Did you make headway on those crow's-feet or bring that redness under control?

Under "No Change," please note anything that you feel continues to need attention and improvement. This is the kind of list a fussy pessimist would make. Be critical.

Improvements   No Change

_____   _____

_____   _____

_____   _____

_____   _____

_____   _____

If you have seen some improvements, you should feel a sense of accomplishment. You did it yourself, without rushing out to a cosmetic dermatologist or a plastic surgeon. And you probably did it without spending a fortune. In many ways, these are my greatest hopes for my campers: self-reliance, independent thinking, empowered consumption, effective skills, and success.

That said, you may not want to rest on your Beauty Camp laurels just yet. An important part of a successful skin-care regimen is occasional experiments with upgrading. Once you've found an ingredient that works for you and doesn't cause irritation, it isn't a bad idea to see if your skin could tolerate a higher strength for even better results.

For example, if you're using a glycolic acid product, take a look at the product label—specifically, the ingredient list. Does the glycolic acid appear somewhat far down the list? If so, I wonder if a slightly stronger solution could have a more dramatic impact on your skin.

CAMP ACTIVITY #2
STEP UP TO THE NEXT LEVEL

From your revamped skin-care regimen, choose the products that you feel have helped the most. Given the time and money that you've invested, you want to know what's working—and what isn't. (I'm curious to know myself! Feel free to write me via my Web site, www.drloretta.com.)

Look at the label of each product, and make a list of the ingredients that you know have some skin-care benefit—things like glycolic acid, salicylic acid, peptides, and hydroquinone. (If you need a refresher course in My Favorite Ingredients, refer back to Week #2.) One product may have multiple active or effective ingredients. Be sure to write down all of them.

With list in hand, you're going to head back to the drugstore or department store and shop for products with similar ingredients but in stronger formulations. For example, if you've been using 1 percent salicylic acid, then move up to 2 percent.

Since you're just experimenting with the stronger formulations at this point, try to avoid buying an entire jar or bottle of a product. Request free samples, or scout around for trial or travel sizes. If you have no choice but to go full size, perhaps you can split the cost with a friend or a fellow Beauty Camper.

Here are some ingredient upgrades that you may want to consider.

Glycolic acid: The products available in drugstores and department stores are up to 10 percent glycolic acid. (They probably are diluted as well.) If you've been using a weaker formulation, you might step up to a 10 percent product. For the first few days, I'd recommend rinsing off the glycolic acid after 20 minutes. Then you can try leaving it on your face.

If you already are using 10 percent glycolic acid, you might switch to a pure glycolic acid product. These "physician-strength" formulas are sold only through doctors' offices. They don't require a prescription, however, so you should be able to place an order online or by phone.

Salicylic acid: If you're using a 0.5 percent product, go to 1 percent; if you're using 1 percent, go to 2 percent—the strongest salicylic acid formulation available for the face without a prescription. A new prescription product called Salex is 6 percent salicylic acid; it's intended to treat thick skin on the elbows and soles of the feet, as well as very flaky skin on the legs.

Hydroquinone: The maximum nonprescription strength for a hydroquinone formulation is 2 percent, so your best bet is to pair it with a retinol product. You could go from 2 percent hydroquinone to a 3 percent prescription product called Melanex. And if 3 percent doesn't produce the desired improvements within 2 to 3 months, you can ask your dermatologist for a 4 percent formulation.

With any of these upgrades, I suggest doing the half-face test, which you may remember from Week #3. Continue with your current regimen on the right side of your face, while using the ramped-up version on the left side. You should see a difference on the left side within a week. Pay attention to any signs of irritation or redness or the sensation of a mild sunburn. If it isn't so bad that it's uncomfortable, then I would try applying the new regimen to your entire face. Give it a week to see what happens. If you continue to see improvement and any irritation or redness hasn't gotten worse, then you know it's time to step up to this next level of skin care.

CAMP ACTIVITY #3
EXFOLIATION, OR PUTTING THE PEDAL TO THE METAL

Enhanced exfoliation is a good idea for any Beauty Camper who is seeking more dramatic results from her skin-care regimen. This could be as simple as switching from washing your face with your hands to using a washcloth or a gentle Buf-Puf. As long as you're sweeping away dead skin cells and clearing pores, almost any ingredient will stand a better chance of working.

On her last visit to her dermatologist, a friend of mine observed that the doctor's skin appeared far smoother than hers, even though they're the same age. The doctor's explanation? He shaves his face every day.

Can shaving off the dead skin-cell layer (the stratum corneum) really help keep your skin smooth and wrinkle free? I will comment on this only as an observer, because I have never felt the urge to shave my face. But it is unusual to see a man with wrinkles in his beard area, even if they appear elsewhere on his face. Men who work outdoors their whole lives, and therefore should have significant sun damage, seldom develop wrinkles where they shave. Men aren't prone to lip lines, either.

In my opinion—and I'm not alone in this—shaving is a form of exfoliation that rejuvenates the skin. As you'll remember from Week #3 of Beauty Camp, exfoliation involves the removal of that outermost dead skin-cell layer, which is precisely what shaving does. Indeed, some doctors use a scalpel blade to gently shave a female patient's face before applying a peel. So for those women who are brave enough to try it, shaving could be an inexpensive but effective method for boosting the exfoliating step of their skin-care regimens.

For years, the most popular method of exfoliation was a peel—an in-office treatment in which the dermatologist would apply an acid to the facial skin. Typically, the patient would develop unsightly scabs, leaving her housebound for 3 to 5 days after the procedure.

Eventually, traditional peels gave way to so-called acid washes—applying a milder acid such as glycolic in multiple (usually weekly or biweekly) sessions. Though achieving results took longer, the patient did not experience as much discomfort or downtime.

Now there are special exfoliating peels that you can apply yourself at home. You'll see them while you're browsing drugstore shelves and department-store cosmetics counters. Some of these products are labeled as acne treatments, while others are for wrinkles. But they are very similar in their ingredients, usually containing glycolic or salicylic acid. Some peels even come with their own brushes, so they're easy to use.

Whichever peel you choose, my only caveat is that you carefully follow the directions provided by the manufacturer.

Please don't experiment with leaving strong acids on your face longer than is recommended. Peels work by causing a chemical reaction on your skin that prompts the shedding of cells. It would be far better to repeat the treatment at the recommended intervals than to risk irritation so severe that you'll look like a burn victim for a week or more. Also, if you're planning to spend time outdoors after your treatment, be sure to apply a generous coat of a zinc-based sunscreen to protect your sensitive skin.

Another option for enhanced exfoliation is at-home microdermabrasion. Many reputable skin-care brands have gotten into the dermabrasion act, selling creams with microdermabrasion particles as well as handheld machines that polish off the dead skin-cell layer. Both of these products are gentler versions of a dermatologist's machine. Many of the microdermabrasion (sometimes called microbuff) creams contain aluminum oxide particles—the same particles often used at dermatologists' offices and day spas.

For in-office microdermabrasion, the dermatologist rubs aluminum oxide crystals (like fine sand particles) over the face, applying constant pressure. I particularly like this treatment for my own face; when I describe it to patients, I compare it to an intense buffing of the skin.

By stripping away the outer, dead skin-cell layer, microdermabrasion improves and evens skin tone. It also minimizes the appearance of fine lines and scars. After using one of these products, please be very gentle to your skin, as it will be more sensitive than ever. Use the gentlest "calming" cleanser you can find, and follow up with a few dabs of a zinc-based sunscreen to help cool and calm your skin.

CAMP LESSON
TROUBLESHOOTING YOUR REGIMEN

It's hard for me to hear about the "No Change" side of your list. I feel as though I have failed you in some way; perhaps I haven't given you the best advice. Maybe you've struggled to follow through on practicing the facial exercises or getting more sleep. I encourage you to make a stronger effort on both fronts. But really, even without doing those things faithfully, you should be seeing fairly significant improvement as long as you've got a great skin-care regimen. So stick with me. All of us have UEs that are stubborn and hard to fix.

Before we dissect your regimen and decide where to fine-tune, I must ask: Could your attitude be part of the problem? Have you been pessimistic from the start of Beauty Camp? It's okay if you have been; some people are pessimistic by nature, and this can be hard to change. My only hope is that you won't allow it to derail your efforts to restore your skin to its healthy, vibrant, youthful glory.

Do you find yourself thinking that skin-care products "are all the same" and "never work" or that you might be beyond help? None of this is true. If you haven't seen significant improvement with your revamped skin-care regimen, then it just isn't strong enough. You can find products that are better suited to your needs. Believe me.

Then again, sometimes the problem is not so much pessimism as a lack of discipline. How faithfully have you been following your skin-care regimen, and how carefully did you choose your products? Did you read the product directions, and are you following them? These things matter over time.

As we move forward, please be mindful of your attitude and your level of commitment. The last thing I would want you to do is to sabotage your own face! There really is no point in spending time with this book and spending money on skin-care products if you aren't going to at least make an effort to get the results you deserve.

GETTING ON TRACK

Now let's go back to your actual skin-care regimen. If your face has not shown the level of improvement that you expected by now, then we need to reconsider everything about your regimen—the products, the strengths, the frequency with which you use them. (This might be a good time for a quick review of Weeks #3 and #4.)

Could your salicylic acid or glycolic acid be too mild? Then you definitely should think about upgrading, as we discussed earlier. Are you using peptides? Are you diligent about exfoliating? If you haven't noticed much change in any age spots or discolorations, then you probably should try a stronger hydroquinone preparation, perhaps in combination with glycolic acid.

Some of the UEs on your "No Change" list might be more difficult to fix than others, especially with at-home treatments. I suspect this is the real issue for most Beauty Campers. Each of the following UEs requires a little extra effort and probably the addition of a new skin-care product.

- Lip lines
- Deep nasolabial folds

- Marionette lines
- Furrowed brow
- Crow's-feet
- Prunelike or "cobblestone" chin

All of us can identify things about our faces that we'd like to change or, even better, make disappear completely. They're kind of like alien life forms; they just don't *belong* here. Other things really don't bother us all that much. They're like old friends; we're accustomed to them, and they're part of our lives. They're the UEs that we can live with.

Just because I have identified certain UEs as stubborn doesn't mean that they must be fixed. As I've said many times and in many ways, our UEs can give us individuality, character, and perhaps a little polish. Just like a house, a face looks more beautiful when it's lived in.

Targeting Your Uninvited Elements

Let's suppose that you have a UE or two that you'd like to do something about. Or you're fine with it now, but down the road . . . who knows? I'll present the best options for treating the most common skin-care dilemmas here. If and when you decide to follow my suggestions, you should start to see improvement in a week or two.

Lip lines: Smokers are prone to lip lines from repeatedly pursing their lips. If you smoke, you should seriously consider quitting—for your skin and for your general health. Drinking through straws or directly out of bottles uses the same muscle above the lip and can aggravate lip lines, too. It may seem silly, but it's a medical and anatomical fact.

My personal pick for treating lip lines is a neuropeptide product. It helps smooth out the lines and, as a bonus, gives a bit of fullness to the lips. If you apply the neuropeptide 3 nights a week, in combination with Retin-A Micro or another retinol product of about 0.15 percent strength, you should notice a difference in your lip lines within about 2 weeks.

If you don't want to wait that long, you can see results more quickly by adding a microdermabrasion product to your skin-care regimen. Look for a microbuff cream containing aluminum oxide crystals and massage it around your lip area for 2 to 3 minutes twice a week. Be gentle, and proceed cautiously until you know how well your skin tolerates this kind of abrasive action. Thoroughly rinse off the cream with tepid water when you're through.

Also apply a peptide-based cream to your lip lines every morning, and use a retinol product—either a retail brand or physician-strength formula—every night. Until you have developed a tolerance for retinol, do not use it immediately before or after microdermabrasion. It will virtually guarantee you a case of irritated skin. If your lips feel sunburned when you apply retinol every night, cut back to every other night. If that doesn't help, cut back to twice a week.

Nasolabial folds and marionette lines: Back in Week #1, we talked about the anatomy of the skin and how deep lines can form on our faces as the skin's fibers and substance begin to break down. Because of the depth of these lines, they really are best described as grooves.

One kind of facial groove is the nasolabial folds, the creases that run from the corners of the nose to the corners of the mouth. They're common among people who have lost a lot of weight quickly or who were very thin to begin with. Some people are prone to them because of the facial structure they inherited.

Marionette lines—another kind of groove—form at the edges of the mouth and run down toward the chin. They look almost like a permanent frown. I like to joke with patients that they can get rid of marionette lines or nasolabial folds by gaining 50 to 75 pounds. Fortunately, that's not the only "treatment." Certain topical products can help reduce these grooves, though they probably won't go away completely.

A brand-name retinol product can be very helpful, especially if you pair it with a leave-on glycolic acid product. Again, exfoliation is a must; at the very least, an at-home peel or a microdermabrasion cream can enhance the effectiveness of the rest of your skin-care regimen and lend a smoother appearance to the skin. I've seen solid improvements in facial grooves when patients use a microbuff cream along with a retinol product.

Furrowed brow: Fixing this UE is notoriously difficult, but many women have seen improvement with a few simple at-home treatments. The first thing that I would try is a neuropeptide product. An at-home peel also could help, as could a stronger leave-on glycolic acid product. Look for pure (undiluted) 10 percent glycolic acid, ideally in a wash-off gel. Apply it for 20 to 30 minutes every other day until your skin becomes accustomed to it. Then step up treatments to every day. If you don't notice any irritation, you might try applying this stronger glycolic acid product in the morning and leaving it on all day, underneath a peptide moisturizer.

Another effective strategy for treating a furrowed brow is to step up exfoliation between the eyebrows. Carefully apply a microbuff cream to the area—though try not to use it on the same day you use glycolic acid gel when you're starting out. Your skin needs time to calm down between treatments. Just 2 minutes twice a week is enough at first. Eventually your skin will adjust to the stronger products. Then gradually work toward 3 to 4 minutes of microdermabrasion, three or four times a week. Just remember to be very gentle when applying the microbuff cream.

You also might want to try a retinoid product, which can be helpful for a furrowed brow. Begin with a brand-name or physician-strength retinol product; if you see good results, you might ask your doctor for something stronger, like Retin-A or Tazorac. Though these are prescription products, getting them may not require a doctor's visit, especially if you're an established patient of the dermatologist.

Crow's-feet and prunelike chin: For these UEs, I would follow the above instructions for at-home treatment of a furrowed brow and facial grooves. Because crow's-feet appear in an especially sensitive area, please take extra care to exfoliate as gently as possible. With consistent use of the recommended products, delicate crow's-feet can decline in number, if not disappear completely.

As for the retinol or prescription retinoid product, start with applications 2 nights a week and increase to every other night. Your skin might not tolerate more than that. If it can take more, ramp up to every night.

I also suggest using a leave-on moisturizer with a strong glycolic acid as an ingredient. The glycolic might cause a tingling sensation. A tingle is good; a sting isn't.

SCARY CAMP STORY:

CALLING IT QUITS

If a product is really irritating or otherwise causing trouble for your skin, don't be afraid to give up on it. I am always surprised and saddened by how many women put up with red, inflamed skin because they won't stop using something that a physician or salesperson recommended.

This happened just recently, when a gorgeous woman—who looks 15 years younger than her chronologic age of 45—came into my office with red, puffy circles under her eyes. They had appeared about 3 months earlier, when another doctor had started her on a prescription retinoid. Even though the product irritated her skin, she believed that if she persevered, her skin would become more tolerant of it (which can happen with glycolic acid and other acid products). But her skin had other ideas.

Thinking this woman felt committed to her retinoid, I explained that if she was happy with the results otherwise, she should try applying the product about an hour before bedtime. That way it wouldn't rub directly onto her pillowcase and, from there, into the skin around her eyes (where she hadn't originally been putting it).

But when I mentioned that she could quit using the retinoid altogether, her face positively lit up. She was so relieved!

All of us need to become more empowered about our skincare regimens, basing them on our own needs and tolerances rather than other people's opinions and advice. If a product isn't working for you, believe me, you can find another one that will.

LAST CAMP ACTIVITY!
BEING HAPPY WITH HOW YOU LOOK

By now you should have a nice-size collection of photos from your time at Beauty Camp. Some were taken at the very beginning of camp, before you knew the difference between a static line and a dynamic line. Some were taken 2 weeks ago, shortly after you'd started using your new-and-improved skin-care regimen, and you were examining your skin tone. Some were taken last week, when you were contemplating changes to your hairstyle and makeup.

I want you to study all of your photos, in order. This is a time for reflection and honesty. Are you happy with what you see? If not, why not? Could your disappointment be rooted in some larger issue in your life? Were you hoping that a dramatic transformation in your appearance might compensate for other disappointments and losses?

I sincerely hope that over the last 5 weeks of Beauty Camp, you've grown happier with your face. After all, *it's your face*. It's the sum of the choices you have made and will make. To embrace your face is to accept who you are, where you've been, where you're going, and what you want from life. To embrace your face is, ultimately, to find peace.

At the end of this book, you'll find a special section called Beauty Camp Extra, where I explore the state-of-the-art in in-office skin treatments and procedures. It's for any camper who's curious to know all that's out there in the realm of cosmetic dermatology. I do hope that before you rush to a doctor's office for Botox injections or laser therapy, you'll give my at-home treatments a fair shake. You may not see significant changes in your most stubborn UEs for another week or two. Patience is a virtue!

If you like what you see now, you'll be even happier with what you see a month from now. Then I invite you to take one more photo of yourself . . . smiling.

Week #6 Review

- *Ramp up, don't give up, your skin-care regimen.*
- *Commit to regular, consistent use of products you believe in.*
- *Study your most stubborn UEs. Which ones do you want to fix, and which ones can you live with?*
- *Know when to give up on a product.*
- *Remember the five Survival Basics: Cleanse, exfoliate, moisturize, rejuvenate, and protect.*
- *Get more sleep!*
- *Do those facial exercises!*
- *Learn to love your face, no matter what.*
- *Smile.*

Epilogue
Good-Bye from Dr. Loretta

Through the 6 weeks that we've spent together at Beauty Camp, I hope that my message of independent thinking and self-reliance and my philosophy of self-respect have come through. I truly believe that every face is beautiful and becomes more so with the passage of time. Defining and embracing your own beauty at every stage of life is the true foundation of sensational skin.

This doesn't come naturally for everyone. Some of us need to think about it and really work at it. We need to find ways to be content with and comfortable in our own skin.

It's funny. When we were younger, we couldn't wait to be older. Children want to be bigger kids. Bigger kids yearn to be adolescents. Teenagers can't wait to be adults. Then sometime around our 40th birthdays, if not sooner, we look in the mirror and fantasize about reclaiming our youth. Somehow it's easier to look back than to look ahead 10, 20, 30 years.

I invite you to think about your next stage and what you will be like when you get there. You know, if you're lucky, one day you will end up old. You'll celebrate your 70th or 80th birthday

. . . or even your 90th or 100th. No matter how many candles you have on your birthday cake, your age is what you make it.

When I was a girl, older women really looked like grannies. They wore formless dark dresses and heavy shoes and pulled their hair back in buns. They didn't update their hairstyles, much less color their hair. Thankfully, times have changed, as have our cultural attitudes and expectations about aging. Older women—and men—don't look as old as they once did. Because of this, we may feel pressure to look even younger than we are.

Yet all of us have seen women who've tried to turn back the clock a bit too far. Their faces seem, well, unnatural. They make us wonder where to draw the line between maintaining our youth and aging gracefully.

I'm 53 now. I can say, honestly, that my sense of self-worth is not completely bound up in my appearance. And yet my appearance definitely matters to me. It can affect how I feel about my day and the world around me. It's clear to me that when I look my best—my face healthy and vibrant, my smile bright—my patients and colleagues, and even my family, respond to me in a more positive way.

It's hard to know how much we should care about our looks. That's the bottom line, isn't it? Maybe it's time to settle into your skin-care regimen and shift your focus to getting more exercise or improving your diet. Your appearance is important, but at the end of the day, many other things are more vital to your general health and well-being.

As you prepare to leave Beauty Camp, I hope that I've empowered you to take charge of your Uninvited Elements (UEs)—to accept and love the ones that don't bother you all that much and to improve the ones that do. Each of us needs to draw her own line—to decide how much we're willing to change and how far we're willing to go to achieve "beauty," however we define it. As a dermatologist and a woman, I've been able to help patients—and family members and friends—make these decisions for themselves. They've found a balance that they can live with and afford. Perhaps now you can do the same.

I hope that you feel more knowledgeable about the skin-care products and procedures currently available, so you can navigate the drugstore aisles and department-store displays with confidence. (Please feel free to tell me what has worked for you and what hasn't, via my Web site: www.drloretta.com.) I hope, too, that you might pass along some of the wisdom of Beauty Camp to your family and friends. In particular, I encourage you to share this guide with your daughters (and sons), who—if they begin a sensible skin-care regimen while they're young, certainly by their teens and twenties—might have far fewer UEs to deal with as they get older.

Mostly, I hope that you'll leave Beauty Camp with a renewed interest in and excitement about your appearance—which might banish even the slightest sense of resignation that can come with time and age. It's never too late to try something new or to see ourselves in a fresh, inspired way.

At the end of the day, I suppose, it's only our attitude that needs to go to Camp. We grow so accustomed to looking at our faces in the mirror that we fail to notice the wonderful person looking back.

—*Dr. Loretta*

THE BEAUTY CAMPER'S
CODE OF CONDUCT

1. I will wash my face with tepid water.

2. I will get 30 extra minutes of sleep every night.

3. I will do my facial exercises.

4. I will go an extra day without shampooing my hair.

5. I will use a clean washcloth every day—and I will launder it in All Free Clear laundry detergent.

6. I will sleep on a 400-thread-count, all-cotton pillowcase.

7. I will read the ingredient lists on skin-care products carefully.

8. I will remember the five Survival Basics: Cleanse, exfoliate, moisturize, rejuvenate, and protect.

9. I will create a daily skin-care regimen and stick with it.

10. When appropriate, I will share skin-care products with family members, friends, and fellow Beauty Campers. This is a Beauty Camp tradition!

11. I will be diligent about researching dermatologists and in-office skin treatments before committing to them.

12. I will remember to look at my face in the mirror as I would at an old friend—with a smile.

Beauty Camp Extra
Inside the Doctor's Office

This week's agenda: Empowering Beauty Campers to find the right doctor and get the right cosmetic treatment—without spending too much money in the process.

Let's begin this post–Beauty Camp session with a question: What brings you here?

- You're a diehard—one of those campers who can't call it quits. Your wherewithal for cosmetic treatments and your desire to improve your appearance keep you on the prowl for the latest and best options.
- You have special skin-care needs and demands. For example, if your job puts you in the public eye on a regular basis, taming your Uninvited Elements (UEs) could be critical to your livelihood.
- You have one particularly stubborn UE—such as a furrowed brow, lip lines, or acne scars—that won't disappear

with at-home treatments (though I hope you've given your ramped-up skin-care regimen time to work).

- You've looked into cosmetic surgery and seriously considered having something pulled or lifted. But you're uncertain about which procedure you should try first. (The funny thing about cosmetic surgery these days: Six months after they've had it, many of my patients return to me for injections or other "booster" treatments.)

- Then again, you might be one of those campers who have always known that cosmetic surgery will never be an option—but cosmetic dermatology treatments are.

- You're just the tiniest bit vain and determined to keep your skin as smooth and clear as possible for as long as possible.

For any of these reasons, or perhaps something else, you're looking for skin-care advice beyond what you've learned during the 6 weeks of Beauty Camp. This session is just for you. We'll discuss the very latest in-office treatments, from Botox injections and collagen fillers to microdermabrasion and Thermage. With the information here, you'll be able to choose the right treatment for your UEs—and your budget. Or you might simply think about what's available, so you can do some planning for the future. The choice is yours!

PLUMP, DON'T PULL

These days, cosmetic surgery seldom is the first—or best—option for correcting UEs. Some faces just aren't well served by the severe pulling of a face-lift or an eye job (*blepharoplasty*, in medical lingo). If your face is thin or your mouth and chin areas aren't full and fleshy, then you definitely are not an ideal candidate for a face-lift. Keep in mind, too, that any asymmetrical elements of the face—such as one eye being larger than the other—can be exaggerated by pulling.

Besides, it's great to have other treatments available to you. Cosmetic surgery comes with a good deal of downtime, expense, and risks—and not everybody is comfortable with it. In the old days, the only option for correcting a sagging or furrowed brow was a surgical procedure called a brow lift. These days, many more patients are choosing Botox injections, which have made the brow lift almost obsolete. Likewise, the conventional face-lift is giving way to high-tech treatments such as Thermage, which uses a high-intensity radio frequency to create a similar "pull" on the skin. (I'll say more about Thermage shortly.)

Before you choose a cosmetic treatment, of course, you need to pinpoint the UE that you're trying to address. You don't want to pursue a certain procedure just because it's new or your dermatologist happens to have the necessary equipment. Tell me your concerns, and I'll help identify the available treatments for them. Then we can concentrate on finding a doctor with the proper training and skills to help you.

A qualified doctor is critical to successful cosmetic treatment. These days, many procedures are performed by both dermatologists and cosmetic surgeons. But within these disciplines, there's tremendous variation in the level of expertise and the availability of equipment. For example, a general dermatologist may specialize in skin cancer and not have much experience with cosmetic treatment. There's no point in wasting this person's time—or yours—on your furrowed brow or lip lines. A skilled cosmetic surgeon may not be all that familiar with the use of Restylane to plump up nasolabial folds, the deep creases that radiate from nose to mouth.

To quickly recap: If you're contemplating cosmetic treatment, your best course of action is to (1) identify your UEs; (2) narrow down to the appropriate procedures, based on your lifestyle, budget, and other factors; and (3) find a doctor with the expertise and experience to administer your procedure of choice.

My UEs—And What I Do about Them

If I were to make a list of my own UEs that I've not been able to correct to my satisfaction with at-home treatments, it would shape up something like this.

- Sagging brow
- Prunish chin
- Puckering around my mouth

Let's start with my sagging brow. Though it's been my most bothersome UE for years, I have never been tempted to fix it with a surgical lift. Then, in 2002, I happened to attend an all-day seminar on new Botox techniques, sponsored by the American Academy of Dermatology. That was my introduction to the Botox brow lift.

After the seminar, I decided to become my first patient, performing the brow lift on myself. The treatment involves a series of four to six Botox injections spaced evenly along the expanse of the upper forehead, just a tad under the hairline. It takes only a few minutes to perform and several days to a week to become effective. Typically, the results last for 4 to 6 months. Once the brow starts to droop again, you repeat the treatment.

I can guess what you're thinking: *Botox?!* Lots of women, including many of my friends, would never dream of getting a Botox injection. And believe me, I'm not here to suggest that every Beauty Camper—or friend of mine—needs one. But from my experience with other cosmetic treatments, nothing equals Botox in effectiveness and safety for correcting a sagging or furrowed brow.

I would caution that the Botox brow lift is a quite advanced procedure that should be performed only by a physician with extensive training and clinical practice in administering the injections. And Botox injections aren't cheap: A brow lift can run anywhere from $300 to $500. But, as I mentioned, it takes exactly 2 minutes, and there's no downtime afterward. By comparison, a surgical brow lift costs between $3,000 and $5,000, and the recovery period can be significant.

When I talk with my patients about Botox injections, many are under the impression that other skin-rejuvenating treatments, such as photofacials and lasers, have been in use longer and therefore have better track records for safety. The truth is, this sort of equipment is changing constantly. Think how quickly personal computers become obsolete as smarter, faster, more sophisticated models take their place. The same holds true for lasers and other treatment devices.

My patients are often surprised when they learn that Botox and other cosmetic injections have been around for more than a decade. They continue to be the treatment of choice for many cosmetic dermatologists. We have become very adept at perfecting our techniques with these injectables and treating patients with a level of expertise and skill rarely seen with other procedures.

As a voluntary professor at the University of Miami who has been teaching residents in cosmetic dermatology how to properly administer injections for 15 years, I do recommend that you try to find a dermatologist who trains other doctors in these procedures. Check at a local medical school or teaching hospital, if you happen to live close to one. Otherwise, look for a physician who is taking classes to stay up-to-date on the latest technology and techniques. I would ask this person whether he or she has tried the treatment on himself or herself.

I do not use any cosmetic injection on a patient that I haven't tried on my own face first—nor is there an injection placement that I haven't considered, reconsidered, and perfected. Beyond the Botox for my sagging brow, I use Restylane to fill out the indented skin of my upper chin—the result of a row of wiggly lower teeth, combined with the bone resorption and fat loss that occur at middle age.

Actually, my chin is my biggest challenge, as it is for many women of a certain age. You probably won't notice this in the flattering (but—I promise you—completely unaltered, unretouched, un–Photoshopped) picture of me on the front cover, but the skin of my lower chin tends to take on a prunish, "cobblestone" appearance. To manage this particular UE, in addition to the products that are part of my skin-care regimen, I've had very good success with injecting just a tiny amount of Botox into the fleshy part of my chin. The cobblestones smooth out almost immediately, and because the injection is in the lower part of my face, its effects last longer—up to 9 months.

The cost of this treatment is about $250—less than for a brow lift because pricing is based on the amount of Botox used. It's very important that the person administering the injection be an expert in the procedure. Otherwise, you could wind up with a droopy lower lip.

High-Tech Choices for Static Lines

Let's go back to one of our earliest camp lessons, in which we explored the differences between static and dynamic lines. Static lines are the ones that are visible on your face even while you are sleeping. They occur with age because of fat loss and sun damage. In older Beauty Campers—women in their seventies and eighties—even dynamic lines can become static over time.

While dynamic lines can become more pronounced with fat loss and sun damage, they are caused primarily by repeated facial movements. Think of the fine creases that form around your eyes when you smile or the deep furrows in your brow when you frown—facial expressions that have given rise to the name *personality lines*. Many smokers develop dynamic lip lines from repeatedly pursing their lips to puff on their cigarettes.

For dynamic lines, one treatment works better than any other: Botox injections. Static lines can be improved and even reversed with a variety of in-office procedures, from peels to photofacials.

Let's focus on cosmetic treatments for static lines. Dermatologists divide these lines into two categories: deep and superficial. We've been discussing them as grooves and fine lines. We'll look at each in turn.

Treatment of Grooves

Some deeper lines on the face occur with the loss of skin substance. Because of their depth, they are best described as grooves rather than lines. Nasolabial folds—the creases that run from the corners of the nose to the corners of the mouth—are one example of a groove. Marionette lines, which create what looks like a perpetual downturn at the corners of the mouth, are another.

By far the most effective way to treat areas like this—which result from the loss of tissue over time—is to fill them. That's why we dermatologists refer to so many of the injections that we administer as fillers. Unlike Botox, which targets the nerves and muscles that create grooves and lines, injections such as collagen and Restylane work by plumping up the skin. This gives the skin a smoother appearance that can last from 2 months to almost a year, depending on the type of filler and the location of the injection.

Fillers are the most immediately satisfying cosmetic treatments that I perform in my office. They not only reduce grooves and fine lines, they also plump up shrinking or naturally thin lips. Restylane injections can fill certain types of acne scars and sometimes chicken pox scars. Lately, I've been using Restylane to help create firmer, better defined jawlines for women whose chins and necks seem to be merging into one. It's also good for filling cheekbones, hands, and other areas.

I believe that for most facial grooves, a properly administered filler is a far better choice than any kind of surgical pull or lift, in terms of outcome. All of us have seen the occasional overzealous face-lift, in which the surgeon seems to have pulled too tightly on the underlying muscles to reduce the depth of grooves. It's true that the grooves may be less noticeable. But the patient ends up looking like she is caught in a windstorm or, even worse, hanging from a hook.

Plump, don't pull. That's my mantra. Adding substance to the underlying skin not only fills in grooves but also reorients the face with a more upward slant, so the person looks as though she's had a bit of a lift. The end result is very aesthetically pleasing: a natural-looking rejuvenation of the face.

There are three kinds of fillers: Restylane, collagen, and autologous fat injections. Each cosmetic dermatologist has his or her favorite, based on his or her success with each. Let's consider each one individually.

Restylane

Restylane is an injection of hyaluronic acid, a substance that's present in all skin. It's capable of holding 1,000 times its weight in water, which helps skin stay plump and hydrated. (Think back to Week #1 of Beauty Camp, when we discussed how skin gets its fullness and firmness from a good fibrous structure and good hyaluronic acid content.)

After an injection of Restylane, the treated area becomes slightly swollen, and the grooves seem instantly corrected. But the euphoria can sink once the patient returns home and most of the swelling subsides. That's when the hyaluronic acid in Restylane begins to soak up water. Before long, the grooves disappear, having been replaced by a smooth, plump surface.

Some patients complain of lumpy skin for several days after receiving Restylane injections. You should be aware that for the first 48 hours or so, the material is very pliable—just like

Silly Putty. I instruct my patients to check their faces the night after treatment—and again the following morning and evening—and gently press down on any area that seems lumpy. The lumpiness should go away. If it doesn't, ask your doctor to examine the area.

The FDA has said that Restylane can be marketed as lasting for at least 6 months, but many of my patients have shown significant improvement for up to 1 year. The key to such long-lasting results is for the doctor to administer enough Restylane at the initial treatment. Often, I'll use two or three syringes at first, and then have the patient return in 2 weeks to see if more injections are necessary. When the person comes in for follow-up many months later, often he or she requires only simple maintenance—a touch-up—which is much less expensive. (A single syringe of Restylane costs between $500 and $750.)

Since being approved by the FDA in January 2004, Restylane has all but replaced collagen injections in most cases. Because it lasts so long and doesn't require any kind of allergy testing, it is my favorite filler.

Zyderm/Zyplast

Both Zyderm and Zyplast are made by Allergan and generally referred to as collagen injections. They have been around for many years and have remained popular among their loyal users.

Both Zyderm and Zyplast are made with collagen extracted from cow skin. The cows are native to the United States; to date, there have been no reports of disease associated with these collagen injections.

Zyderm has been available since 1981. When it first came

Precautions against Bruising

Bruising is common with filler treatments. Some patients come to me solely because they have developed serious bruises after receiving fillers from other doctors. Usually they know someone who came to me for treatment and showed little or no bruising.

I am not suggesting that I am better than my colleagues at administering filler injections. If my patients aren't bruising as much, it is due in part to all of the precautions that I like to take. I suggest that any patient facing a procedure involving multiple injections—including Botox, Restylane, collagen, and autologous fat transplants—take the following precautionary steps.

1. Avoid consuming alcohol for at least 2 days before treatment.

2. Discontinue vitamin E, anti-inflammatory drugs such as Advil and Aleve, and aspirin for 5 days beforehand.

3. If you're taking prescription blood thinners, ask your doctor if you may stop using them for several days before treatment. If not, tell your dermatologist or cosmetic surgeon about them.

out, it met with great fanfare. But soon patients were commenting that the improvements derived from Zyderm didn't last long enough—in some cases, just 6 to 8 weeks. The complaints prompted the manufacturer to develop Zyplast. Because the collagen molecules in Zyplast are cross-linked, the product

4. If you have a low pain threshold, be sure to ask ahead of time for a numbing cream, which will be applied about 45 minutes prior to the injections. Once the cream kicks in, you won't feel the needle being inserted into your skin—which means you're less likely to move during treatment. Movement makes the procedure painful, and it can increase the risk of bruising.

5. Apply ice compresses to the affected skin for 5 to 10 continuous minutes after treatment. If your face is very red or painful when you leave the doctor's office, you can follow up with additional ice compresses for an hour or two after your injections. (This may be necessary with fillers but definitely should not be with Botox.)

6. If you see any bruising whatsoever, ask your doctor about applying a vitamin K cream. Topical vitamin K is excellent at helping to speed the healing of bruises. I keep samples of the cream in my office and give them to any patient who shows signs of bruising post-treatment.

doesn't break down so quickly. The results should last at least 3 months.

Both collagen products require allergy testing at least 1 month prior to treatment. For treatment on the face, two separate allergy tests are ideal. This factor alone makes Restylane—

which can be administered the same day as the first consultation—more appealing to most people. In my practice, I tend to reserve collagen injections for the occasional patient who is extremely thin-skinned and at risk for lumps or bruising, which are more likely with Restylane.

Patients should be very happy with what they see immediately after receiving collagen injections. In fact, I often caution my patients not to spend time studying their faces in the mirror after treatment. They will see improvement, with minimal pain and no real downtime to speak of.

The problem with collagen, I explain, is the unpredictability of what happens next. Sometimes the results just don't last very long. How long is enough? Ideally, a patient will be content with the improvement for 3 to 4 months after the initial treatment. But lots of patients return much sooner for booster treatments.

Collagen comes in several syringe sizes, ranging from 1 to 2.5 cubic centimeters. The fee varies, depending on the amount collagen used; a single treatment generally costs between $300 and $700.

Autologous Fat Injections

This procedure involves extracting a patient's own fat, usually from the thighs or buttocks, and injecting it into the face. The good news: It tends to be cheaper than Restylane or collagen injections because the doctor can take as much fat as needed. The bad news: If you're thin, you may not have that much fat in the "donor" areas. Also, since the procedure essentially is a transplant, some of the fat may not "take," which means the doctor may need to repeat the treatments several times.

Autologous fat injections tend to be more painful than some other injections. They usually cause unsightly swelling and bruising that last for a week or longer, leading to considerable downtime.

If you choose to go the fat injection route, my best advice is to conduct thorough research to find a physician who has performed a lot of these procedures. Expertise on the part of the treating doctor is very important if you hope to have a good outcome.

Ten years ago, I bought all the necessary equipment to perform autologous fat injections. I received rigorous hands-on training, performed five procedures for free—and wasn't happy with the results. I haven't done one since. I always try to attend professional meetings that include presentations on autologous fat injections. It has helped me reach the conclusion that only a select few physicians administer this treatment well, mostly because they have vast experience in it.

Treatment of Acne Scars

It's possible to treat certain types of very deep "ice pick" acne scars with fillers. In order to test this—without having to charge the patient for an expensive filler substance—I will start with an injection of sterile saline into the scar. If the scar lifts, then I will inject one of the approved commercial fillers, usually Restylane.

Sometimes a scar is so deep or so dense and fibrous that the filler can't plump up and smooth out the affected skin. In such cases, it may be worthwhile to have the scar cut out and stitched together with fine sutures. This should be done only by a physician with expertise and experience in scar revision surgery.

To Plump or Not to Plump

A lower lip tends to look very nice and naturally beautiful if it is plumper than the upper lip (ideally, by about 50 percent). Many women do want fuller lips—and if you've perused any beauty magazines lately, you know that lip enhancement is appealing even to twentysomethings.

If you're contemplating this sort of procedure for yourself, please work closely with your doctor to make sure that your lips stay in proper proportion. Don't get an injection in your upper lip and neglect your lower lip. I'm afraid you could wind up looking like you've suffered a terrible bee sting!

Years ago, lip enhancement didn't last that long, so any mistakes went away quickly. Now that most dermatologists have made the switch to Restylane, you could be stuck with poorly proportioned lips for 6 months or more.

Treatment of Fine Lines

In most cosmetic dermatology practices, the mainstay treatments for fine lines are peels and microdermabrasion. But they're not your only options. Certain types of fine lines will improve quite nicely with filler agents.

A great many of my patients are happy with using Restylane for lip lines. It lasts longer than collagen and remains in place, even creating a nice edge or border around the lips. This can help keep your lipstick from bleeding.

Of the two collagen fillers, Zyderm is thinner than Zyplast, but it lasts a considerably shorter time. It can become prohibitively expensive for patients to return as often as necessary for booster treatments.

Many physicians are not happy with the prospect of choosing between a product that will cause lumpiness and one that won't last long enough. I've gotten the best results by injecting Restylane right at the rim of the upper lip. Since the filler isn't going directly into the lip lines, there's less risk of lumpiness posttreatment.

Microdermabrasion and Peels

The state of the art in in-office exfoliation has moved beyond the traditional chemical peel. Cosmetic dermatologists offer a range of exfoliating procedures that produce good results with very limited downtime or discomfort.

All forms of exfoliation strip away the stratum corneum, the dead layer of cells that sits on the surface of the skin. Generally, the two most popular exfoliants are microdermabrasion and peels.

Microdermabrasion involves the use of a mechanical device to rub abrasive particles—often aluminum oxide or salt crystals—under constant pressure against the skin. This not only helps erase fine lines, it also evens skin tone and reduces the appearance of scars.

For a peel, the doctor applies an agent—typically acidic—to the skin to cause a chemical injury. This prompts the skin to begin shedding any dead, injured cells. The process takes several days.

One type of peel, known as the *TCA peel*, has been around

since at least the 1970s. TCA is shorthand for *trichloroacetic acid*, a relatively strong acid in concentrations of 15 to 35 percent. When applied to the skin, TCA almost immediately creates a "frosted" appearance. As this frosting develops, the patient feels a burning sensation that is anywhere from minimally to moderately uncomfortable. Ideally, the doctor will instruct the patient to begin applying ice compresses as soon as the frosting sets in. The ice will relieve the discomfort, but it will not dilute the acid or otherwise interfere with treatment.

The advantage of the TCA peel is that the patient can expect quite noticeable improvement, provided she is a good candidate and the treating doctor has received thorough training in the procedure. The two obvious disadvantages are the discomfort and the amount of downtime associated with the TCA peel. After treatment, the patient generally can't resume normal activities for anywhere from 3 to 7 days. She also must avoid the sun entirely for at least 2 months posttreatment. In fact, most dermatologists agree that it isn't safe to perform TCA peels during summer because of the possibility of a patient getting inadvertent sun exposure. This can lead to prolonged redness and, later, postinflammatory hyperpigmentation (staining of the skin).

I cannot overemphasize the importance of good patient selection in the safe use of the TCA peel. If your skin is prone to developing dark spots after an injury such as a bug bite or kitchen burn, you probably would not do well with a TCA peel. In fact, some patients develop stains because of injury to the skin that occurs during the procedure itself.

At the University of Miami School of Medicine, I have taught the resident physicians in the cosmetic dermatology clinic how to perform the TCA peel. In the past several years, we have all but stopped this practice, because the newer peels are so much safer. That said, if for any reason you want a deeper, TCA-type peel, please be sure to get it from a qualified physician who has performed many of them—and who's willing to spend time discussing the procedure and its outcomes with you before moving ahead.

Among the alternatives to the TCA peel is the *glycolic acid peel*, or *glycolic wash*. The word "wash" alludes to the fact that the doctor rinses off the acid at the end of the procedure, which abruptly stops further reaction with the skin. The procedure involves no actual peeling, so patients can return to their normal activities immediately after treatment. The glycolic wash doesn't produce the dramatic immediate improvement of the TCA peel, but most patients seem willing to wait for results in exchange for greater safety and less downtime.

One definite advantage of the glycolic wash is its versatility. The acid can be left on for as little as 1 minute or as long as 15 minutes, making the procedure tolerable for those patients with the most sensitive skin while extending the leave-on time for others, so they might see faster results. Another plus: For patients who developed redness or staining as an outcome of a previous, stronger peel, the glycolic wash can help correct any persistent discoloration of the skin.

The only precautions with a glycolic wash are to wear sunscreen before and after treatment and to not apply makeup for 1 hour afterward (though generally, patients who don't have sensitive skin and don't want to return to their normal activities without makeup should be okay to put on their "faces"). Also, if you're using an exfoliant or another potentially irritating

Speak Up about Cold Sores

If you are prone to cold sores near your mouth, be sure to tell your doctor before undergoing any injection or peel. He or she can give you some herpes-suppression pills at the time of the procedure and send you home with more. (Cold sores are caused by the herpes simplex virus.) Actually, taking Valtrex—the best of the herpes-suppression medications—is an absolute must before any cosmetic treatment around your mouth. If you don't take the medication before or immediately after treatment, you run the risk of a terrible outbreak.

product in your at-home skin-care regimen, I recommend not applying the product for a day (or night) or two after treatment.

Lasers and More

At about the time interest in the TCA peel waned, another cosmetic treatment rose to take its place. It's known as *laser resurfacing*, and it involves the programmed burning of the skin surface to reduce or eliminate fine lines.

Laser resurfacing grew in popularity in the 1990s, in part because it could be performed on distinct "anatomic units"—such as the area around the eyes or mouth—in addition to the whole face. At first, the lasers were much stronger, with the carbon dioxide laser becoming the most popular. Although so-called laser ablation produced dramatic results in some cases, it also caused tremendous pain, prolonged redness, considerable downtime, and—at worst—permanent scarring.

In contrast to a laser, which has a steadily focused light beam, a newer technique known as *intense pulsed light* (IPL) uses a rapidly flashing light. It's much like the flashbulb of a camera continuously firing—which explains how the procedure earned its alternative name, *photofacial*. IPL is terrific for remodeling collagen and rejuvenating skin, as well as for reducing age spots.

Thermage may be one of the most widely publicized rejuvenation procedures to come our way in recent years. The radio-frequency device received FDA approval in 2003. Some of the early outcomes seemed impressive, but then Thermage was all but written off as too painful and expensive and not especially effective for anyone over 40. At this writing, physicians are experimenting with using the Thermage device on a lower setting to minimize pain. They go over the affected area repeatedly, continuing treatment until they actually see the skin contract, which means they're getting an effective "pull" from Thermage.

High-Tech Choices for Dynamic Lines

I must admit that the first time I saw a TV commercial for Botox, I had no idea what sort of product it was pitching. Yet, like so many viewers, I found the ad totally captivating. I admired the youthful appearance of each model as she revealed that she was in her forties or fifties—or older. I wondered what nutritional supplement or hair-care product, or even makeup line, she was using. Maybe, I reasoned, the ad was for an amazing new diet or piece of fitness equipment. Whatever it was, I wanted it, because I wanted to look more like those women.

Their bodies, their hair, their makeup, their clothing—they had *everything* going for them.

So it came as a disappointment when I finally realized that the ad was for injectable *Botulinum* toxin (marketed as Botox Cosmetic). To me, the FDA's decision to let the manufacturer promote Botox as a treatment for frown lines somehow didn't jibe with the full-body shots of gorgeous models.

Thanks in part to all the advertising, about 60 percent of my new patients ask questions about either Botox or Restylane. Usually these women (and men) want to know which of these aggressively marketed products would do the best job of making them look younger and more attractive—maybe even like the models in the ads. Sometimes they aren't entirely sure just what these products can and can't do. This was driven home to me recently, when a patient asked if Botox could remove the scars from her breast implants. (It can't.)

I know I've said it before, but I can't stress it enough: It's absolutely vital to be an informed consumer—and to not let the excitement and hubbub generated by slick marketing campaigns get the better of you and your common sense. In the same way you need to learn about any skin-care product at the drugstore or department-store cosmetics counter, you need to be smart about the procedures that are available in a dermatologist's or cosmetic surgeon's office—and not leave all of the decision making in the hands of the doctor or the marketers.

Even I needed to do a reality check after watching the commercial for Botox. I drew a deep breath and reminded myself that the injections wouldn't shrink my waistline, so I wouldn't be able to squeeze into the same slick jeans that the model was wearing. Yet for a moment, I got sucked in by what I was seeing—and I'm a dermatologist, so I should know better. The point is, when considering any cosmetic treatment, each of us needs to proceed with intelligence, caution, and skepticism.

Still . . . I must admit that what Botox has done to raise my sagging brow is fantastic. I am totally hooked!

What to Expect from Botox Injections

What is *Botulinum* toxin anyway, aside from the culprit that contaminated cold cuts and caused an outbreak of botulism poisoning years back? The medical benefits of this potentially deadly toxin surfaced more than 2 decades ago, when doctors first injected a diluted form of a protein extracted from *Botulinum* into the muscles of patients with certain eye and neurological diseases. One astute female eye surgeon who used Botox as a treatment in her practice noticed diminished wrinkling around the eyes of patients who were receiving regular injections. The eye surgeon happened to be married to a dermatologist, so the two tested Botox on some staff members and friends. The rest is history.

For those who are weak of heart about having an extract of a bacterium most commonly associated with food poisoning injected into their faces, it's important to note that the protein from *Botulinum* is diluted about 3,000 times to make it safe for cosmetic use. Most patients are relieved to hear that they'd need a sizable dose of Botox—about 28 bottles in one sitting—in order to experience any kind of internal, systemic effect. A typical treatment involves injecting less than half of a bottle.

To erase dynamic lines on the face, a doctor will inject Botox directly into the muscles responsible for the wrinkling. For crow's-feet, for example, treatment would consist of injections at two to four places on each side of the affected area, about 1 centimeter away from the eye socket.

To minimize bruising, the most common side effect of Botox treatment, the patient should not lie down or work out for at least 4 hours afterward. Also, patients respond better to the injections if they exercise the affected muscle group for 5 minutes or so of every waking hour during the first 24 hours posttreatment. So let's suppose that you've received Botox injections for frown lines. You'd want to practice scrunching and then relaxing your brow for 5 minutes every hour. For crow's-feet, you could break into a wide grin and then return to a "neutral" position.

One interesting fact to keep in mind: Botox does not take effect until about 3 to 8 days after treatment. I advise patients to return for a follow-up visit after 2 weeks, to be sure that they've achieved optimal results.

Precautions You Need to Know

Botox has very few possible side effects. When they occur, however, they can be alarming. In the cases on which I've consulted, all of the side effects arose from problems with the injection sites. If you are considering Botox, it might be helpful to have an idea of where *not* to get injections. Here are the problems that can occur—and the precautions that can be taken to avoid them.

For crow's-feet: An injection should be at least 1.5 centimeters from the outermost corner of the eye, the so-called *outer canthus*. If it's closer than that, the patient is at risk for developing *strabismus*, or an involuntary horizontal movement of the eye. Although this side effect generally doesn't last more than several weeks, it should be totally avoidable with proper place-ment of the injections.

At the dermatology clinic where I teach resident physicians how to administer Botox, a 33-year-old woman recently returned after successful treatment of her frown lines and requested injections for her crow's-feet. After talking with this patient, mirror in hand, we explained that she was not a candi-date for treatment. Why? Because all of her lines—which weren't very deep to begin with—were well within 1.5 centi-meters of her eyes. We couldn't place the injections close enough to her crow's-feet to ensure much success in eliminat-ing them.

We advised this patient to slather on sunscreen right up to her eye area. (A chemical-free sunscreen, like zinc oxide or titanium dioxide, will not irritate the eyes.) We also showed her how she could smile just the slightest bit less exuberantly, to avoid repeated creasing around her eyes. When she'd return in 4 to 6 months for booster treatment of her frown lines, she would have minimized her crow's-feet simply by following that advice.

One caution to anyone who's seeking Botox injections for crow's-feet: It's critical to be conservative in treating the lowest lines that make up the "starburst" around the eyes. A very com-petent physician will leave these few lines alone. It's a more aesthetically pleasing approach.

Sometimes, in the interest of thoroughness, a physician will go for all of the lines—upper and lower. In such cases, it's best to use just half the usual dose of Botox at the lowermost injec-tion site on each side. Otherwise, the patient may experience what I call the *girdle effect*. When he or she smiles, an excessive amount of skin bunches up at the point of interface between the treated and untreated areas. It reminds me of how a cellulite-laden thigh looks when it's jammed into tight support hose that reach only a bit above the knee.

This problem also can occur in people who previously underwent a face-lift and are now receiving Botox treatment for crow's-feet. In most cases, the problem is avoidable, provided the physician uses just half the dose in the lowermost injection site.

For a drooping brow: In a brow lift, the physician administers Botox near the top of the forehead (or *frontalis*) muscle. This muscle is responsible for the position of the eyebrows. Injecting Botox several centimeters above the brow line allows the patient to raise her brows, while at the same time giving them a lifted, somewhat arched appearance.

It must be said that some physicians are more skilled than others with the Botox brow lift and get better results. A word of warning, though: If the injections are too close to the eyebrows, it actually can lower the brows instead of lifting them.

For forehead lines: Four or five evenly spaced Botox injections across the width of the forehead should erase any horizontal lines in this area. It's a straightforward and rewarding procedure, especially if you are one of those people who habitually raise their eyebrows every time they open their mouths— and now have a forehead full of very deep grooves (as I have seen even in people in their early thirties).

Should the injections be too close to the upper rim of the eye socket (known as the *superior rim of the orbit*)—generally, within 1.5 centimeters of it—it can lead to *pstosis*. This is the medical term for an inability to fully open the eye. Fortunately, this unwelcome side effect should go away within a matter of weeks, but it can be very bothersome in the meantime.

Avoiding eyelid pstosis is as simple as making sure that your doctor measures how close he or she is to the upper rim before administering an injection. If you have any reservations, don't hesitate to ask your doctor to mark where the injections will go before you get them—though if for some reason you are not 100 percent confident in your doctor, then I must ask: Why are you seeing him or her for treatment?

For frown lines: It still amazes me that as of spring 2006, the treatment of frown lines is the only cosmetic use for which Botox Cosmetic has received FDA approval. All of the other uses we've talked about here are what are known as *off-label*. In other words, doctors can administer Botox for other indications at their own discretion, but the manufacturer cannot market the product for these purposes.

When performed properly, Botox injections are very effective for frown lines. Hundreds of thousands of patients have turned to Botox to "eliminate the 11s," as the ad campaign for the procedure suggests. After treatment, you won't be able to furrow your brow if you try. (You might need to wear sunglasses more often, because you won't be able to squint against the sun's rays, either.)

Some patients who come to me aren't happy with the Botox treatments they received at other doctors' offices. In fact, they simply aren't responding to the injections. The necessary treatment doses to achieve optimal results can vary widely.

For instance, if a patient is athletic and works out regularly, he or she will develop stronger muscles in the frown area. Depending on the intensity of exercise (which is not always so obvious, since the activities can range from lifting weights to biking uphill), the patient could need up to three times the usual dose of Botox. The same is true for people who work outdoors and may squint a lot to avoid getting sun in their eyes. If you are considering Botox injections for your frown lines, be sure to talk with your doctor about these and other lifestyle factors. He or she can adjust the dose as necessary.

For a crepey neck: In the hands of an experienced treating doctor, very small doses of Botox can help erase the horizontal bands that ring the neck. The injections may even tighten the skin in this area. But please, please choose your doctor carefully—and if you can't find one with training and experience in this procedure, then don't do it at all! I've seen what can happen when a physician with inadequate expertise tries to perform this treatment. At best, the results are lackluster if not downright disappointing. In a worst-case scenario, the injection can go too deep into the neck muscles, causing temporary paralysis and an inability to swallow.

SCARY BOTOX STORY

Not long ago, I attended an advanced course in Botox Cosmetic treatment, during which my fellow physicians and I were presented with a particular case. First we were shown a preop photo of a woman who wanted to get rid of some lines around her neck. Next we were shown a postop photo of the same woman—this time, with a plastic tube coming out of her mouth. She had to be fed through the tube for several weeks after receiving Botox injections. The treatment had paralyzed the muscles that allowed her to chew and swallow food.

Thankfully, the patient made a full recovery. But her story underscores the importance of finding a very well trained, experienced physician to administer Botox injections. This is especially true for so-called off-label uses, meaning those that the FDA hasn't approved for that specific purpose.

How Much Can You Expect to Spend?

As you might expect, the pricing of Botox treatments varies greatly, reflecting the wide range in dosages as well as the wide range in cost per unit. Depending on where you live, a unit of Botox can cost between $12 and $15. A frown line may require 20 to 60 units, depending on how muscular the area is.

How much Botox will you need? It depends on your age, skin quality, facial structure, and medical history (in particular, prior cosmetic surgery). It is logical and reasonable to ask your doctor for a cost estimate prior to beginning treatment. That said, if you are comparison shopping and come across a physician who's charging a very low fee, you can be pretty certain that he or she isn't using a dosage that will provide optimal results. The latest scoop on Botox "dosing" is that a small number of units may produce pretty dramatic improvement right after treatment, but the effects won't last long. Generally, the higher the dosage, the better and more durable the results.

I would be remiss if I didn't share with you the anecdotal evidence that I've been collecting by following up with patients who receive Botox injections. Many of them are a decade older since starting treatment, and their lines look better now than 10 years ago. What's the explanation? If you can't use a muscle group day after day, the muscles smooth out, and their associated lines and crinkles disappear.

Do you know someone who seems to have a perpetually angry expression, partly because of extreme strength training? Those bulky frown muscles will lose their identity with continued Botox treatment. My patients with deeply furrowed brows routinely report that, thanks to Botox, their foreheads are smoother at age 50 than at 40.

Finding a Qualified Treating Doctor

Now that you're armed with information about various in-office cosmetic treatments, including the benefits and risks of each, it's time to look for a skilled, experienced physician who can perform the procedures in which you're interested. You might start by contacting your family doctor or local hospital for referrals or by asking family members and friends—and fellow Beauty Campers—for their recommendations. For additional leads, you might pay a visit to the cosmetics counter of an upscale department store and talk with the more seasoned sales personnel. Often these women are in the know.

Once you have a list of names and contact information, you can make calls to the various doctors' offices. If a certain doctor can't take your call, then ask to speak with the physician's assistant or nurse. He or she should be able to answer some basic questions about the doctor's expertise in certain cosmetic treatments.

Be prepared to get specific about what you're seeking treatment for and which procedure you're interested in. Find out whether the doctor has had good success with the UE that you want to fix. Generally, doctors are pretty straightforward with this sort of information. Their answers may range from "Sure!" to "I can help if you have a lot of patience and follow all of my instructions," to "I can try, but don't get your hopes up too high." Other questions that you may want to ask:

- "What's your level of confidence in this treatment?"
- "Will you or someone else on your staff administer the treatment?"
- "What if the treatment doesn't work?"
- "What is the downtime or recovery period?"
- "What's the worst thing that could happen during or after treatment?"
- "What is the cost?"
- "How often will I need booster treatments, and what is their cost?"

Once you think you've found a suitable doctor, I suggest scheduling an appointment for a consultation. Don't forge ahead with the treatment just yet. During the consultation, ask again about this doctor's expertise in the treatment you're considering. Try not to be intimidated by your surroundings, even though you're on the doctor's turf.

If the consultation raises questions about the qualifications or experience of your first-choice doctor, I would not hesitate to seek a second opinion. Many patients come to my office for just this reason. Often they tell me that the staff at the first physician's office seemed more like department-store clerks than clinic personnel, pushing them to purchase hundreds of dollars' worth of skin-care products—and insisting that they'd see real improvement only if they used the entire "system."

If you are considering Botox treatments—and even if you understand all of the downsides and precautions—I would be doubly careful about finding a qualified doctor. I use a good amount of Botox in my practice, but other doctors use even more and have terrific expertise in administering the injections. How do you get this sort of information? One possible resource is www.botoxcosmetic.com. The Web site identifies doctors in your area who buy and use a good amount of Botox in their practices.

The catch is, any doctor can purchase Botox Cosmetic, with or without formal training. Just recently, a nurse contacted me to find out if she could come to my office to watch how I administer Botox injections. It seems that her boss, a cosmetic surgeon, had begun offering Botox treatments to his patients, but he was a little unclear about the proper technique. They had sought guidance from the manufacturer of Botox Cosmetic, asking if anyone could come to the office and provide training. The answer was no. Instead, the manufacturer recommended buying a training video for $200. Ultimately, the surgeon turned over the procedure to his nurse, since he no longer wanted to do it. That's right: It is not uncommon for doctors to have their RNs administer Botox to patients.

Once you've consulted a doctor about your particular UE— and you're satisfied with the recommended course of treatment, benefits and risks, maintenance requirements, and costs—you can go ahead and schedule an appointment for the procedure. Feel free to take time to think about all the information you've gathered before you make a decision to move forward. And if you don't find the right doctor on your first try, keep searching until you do.

Putting Together a
Reasonable Budget

How much can you afford to spend on your appearance? This may seem like a trick question because answering it is so difficult. We want to look our best. We want to address our most pressing UEs. It may seem as though we should spare no expense—especially after reading an entire book on skin care, in which we've learned that all sorts of products and procedures hold tremendous promise. But since none of your UEs are life threatening, is fixing them really worth the expense?

You need to be honest with yourself—and with your spouse or partner, who may be shouldering some of the cost of treatment. Lots of women try to sneak in trips to the dermatologist or cosmetic surgeon, assuming that it won't add up to much in the long run. But it will. Cosmetic treatments can be frightfully expensive—and because they are purely cosmetic, they aren't covered by health insurance.

My advice is to set a budget and then determine just what you can accomplish with it. Think of it as you would a kitchen or bathroom renovation. Be reasonable and practical—but also leave room to fulfill a few dreams along the way.

When calculating how much you can spend on cosmetic treatments, be sure to account for maintenance. Restylane will last 6 to 8 months; Botox, 4 to 6 months—possibly longer, depending on the location of the injections. The booster treatments may not be as expensive, but you should figure on at least one or two a year.

Instead of asking how much you can spend, perhaps a better question is, how *little* can you spend? In other words, which treatment will give you the most benefit for the least cost? It's something to ask your doctor during the initial consultation. The following chart will give you an idea of the going prices for various cosmetic treatments.

U.E.	PROCEDURE	PRICE RANGE
Acne scarring	Microdermabrasion & Restylane injections	$300–$700
Age spots	Intense pulsed light	$500–$1,500
Broken capillaries	V-beam laser	$250–$500
Cobblestone chin	Botox injection every 8–12 months	$150–$250
Crow's-feet	Glycolic peels (6–10) Salicylic peels	$50–$100 each $100–175 each
Furrowed brow	Botox injections every 4–6 months	$300–$500
Lip lines	Restylane injections every 6–8 months	$325–$1,200
Seborhheic keratoses (raised age spots)	Electrodessication	$150–$300
Unwanted hair	Alexandrite laser	$300–$1,000

ONE LAST CAMP STORY

As I was in the final stage of writing this book, a new patient came to see me. A smiling, attractive woman, she explained that the year before, she had attended a silent auction at her children's school, where she'd bid on and won a gift certificate for a Restylane treatment in my office. She'd jumped at the chance, she said, to see a cosmetic dermatologist with such a good reputation. Then she got busy with other things and time passed. In fact, the gift certificate would expire the very next day.

Why did she want a Restylane treatment? She was 55 and the mother of two young children, she explained. When she'd drop off her kids at school, she'd hear other moms—usually 10 to 15 years younger than her—talking about their latest injections, peels, and other cosmetic treatments. Realizing that she was running out of time to use the gift certificate, she finally summoned the courage to make an appointment.

But there was a problem. She really had no idea what Restylane treatment entailed—or what it would do for her. Beyond that, when I took out a mirror to help her assess her own face, she struggled to pinpoint what she was unhappy with and what she'd want to change.

When I asked about her skin-care regimen—whether she'd tried any creams with peptides or alpha hydroxy acids (AHAs) or products with lipids or neuropeptides—she stared at me blankly. It was as though I suddenly had begun talking in some incomprehensible foreign language.

I suggested that she take some candid photos of her face— possibly in front of her bathroom mirror, where she'd have good lighting—to determine whether anything about her face bothered her. I sent her home with samples of products from my own skin-care line, including an exfoliating cleanser, a lipid-laden serum, an AHA cream with peptides, and a zinc-based sunscreen with Colhibin and Elhibin. I also gave her some reading material on Restylane. She could apply the gift certificate—which I extended by 1 month—toward whatever products or treatments would work best for her.

It was an abbreviated version of Beauty Camp, I suppose. This woman deserves to have sensational skin—and I made a sincere promise that I'd do whatever I could to help her reach a decision about what, if anything, she'd want to correct or improve about her appearance. Although you and I may never meet face-to-face, I hope that I've been able to do the same for you.

Good luck in all things—and remember to get more sleep!

A Resource List

New skin-care products and procedures will continue to pop up as time goes on. I hope that you will use the wisdom you've gained through Beauty Camp to investigate their ingredients and track down objective information and data to support product claims. Doing this sort of online research can be enlightening, empowering—and fun.

I invite you to start your online exploration by visiting my Web site, www.drloretta.com. Here you will find up-to-date, reliable information on skin-care ingredients, as well as the products I have been formulating since 1993. Back then, this sort of information seemed very hard to come by. It was frustrating for me not just as a doctor but as a woman on the brink of turning 40. As I looked to the future, I just couldn't imagine myself getting a brow lift, a face-lift, or any of the other cosmetic procedures that I am still avoiding all these years later.

On a day off from work, I literally woke up with the idea that I would formulate my own skin-care products—and that as an experienced dermatologist (and a woman and a rather Gung Ho Beauty Camper), I could create lines for other physicians, as well. To date, I've developed products for more than 1,000 physicians from all over the globe, using a mix of intense research, clinical experience, test results, and patient feedback. I make every effort to select only the most effective, state-of-the-art ingredients and combine them in just the right amounts to produce great results with minimal adverse effects.

Visitors to my Web site can also gain insights into how to address different skin-care needs and find answers to questions that unintentionally haven't received full discussion in this book. The site is easily navigable and uses tips from the book to help Beauty Campers and other clients choose the best products for them.

Beyond my Web site, you can find information on virtually any skin-care ingredient, product, or procedure by entering its name into a search engine such as www.google.com or www.yahoo.com or a metasearch engine such as www.dogpile.com. You also might check out the following Web sites, which offer a wide selection of products and brands, including some that you may not find in drugstores or department stores. Often these sites pick up specialty products and new brands before they're available at retail.

www.blissworld.com

www.dermstore.com

www.drugstore.com

www.platinumskincare.com

www.sephora.com

www.skinplanet.com

www.skinstore.com

The manufacturers of certain skin-care ingredients, products, and equipment have their own Web sites, too. On most you'll find detailed descriptions of the treatments, along with "physician locator" tools that identify by zip code those doctors who offer the treatments. Among the sites that you may find helpful:

www.botoxcosmetic.com

www.novalismedical.com

www.restylaneusa.com

www.thermage.com

FOR YOUR ORIENTATION PHOTOS
(WEEK #1)

FOR YOUR ORIENTATION PHOTOS (WEEK #1)

FOR YOUR ORIENTATION PHOTOS
(WEEK #1)

FOR YOUR CHECK-IN PHOTOS
(WEEK #4)

FOR YOUR CHECK-IN PHOTOS
(WEEK #4)

FOR YOUR CHECK-IN PHOTOS
(WEEK #4)

FOR YOUR "AFTER" PHOTOS
(WEEK #6)

FOR YOUR "AFTER" PHOTOS
(WEEK #6)

FOR YOUR "AFTER" PHOTOS
(WEEK #6)

Index

Underlined page references indicate boxed text.

E

Elastin
  age effect on, 33–34
  Elhibin to prevent breakdown of, 49, 68
Electrodessication, for seborrheic keratoses, 145–46
Elhibin, 49, 68
Epidermis, 33
Estrogen, as cause of
  blood vessel breakage, 154, 156
  skin blotching, 113
Eucerin Redness Relief, 149
Exercise, effect on skin-care regimen, 124
Exfoliation
  benefits of, 103
  enhanced, 190–92
  methods
    glycolic acid, 69–71, 104, 224
    microdermabrasion, 104, 192, 221
    salicylic acid, 80, 104, 192
    scrubbing, 104–6
    shaving, 190–91
    TCA peel, 221–23
    using peels, 191–92
  overdoing, 105, 192
  reasons for, 103, 104
Eyebrows, 177. See also Brow lift
Eyelid pstosis, as Botox side effect, 230–31
Eyeliner, 177–78
Eyeliss, 69, 153–54
Eye makeup, 177–78
Eyes
  analyzing in Orientation photos, 23
  dark circles under, 153–54
  sleep effect on appearance of, 26
Eye shadow, 177

F

Face
  cleansing, 101–3
  water temperature for washing, 88
Face lift
  asymmetrical facial elements, effect on, 208
  as first treatment option, 207–8
Facial exercises
  description, 28–29
  meat-chewing, 30–31
  smiling, 29–30
Fade cream, 131, 136
Fat injections, autologous, 218–19
FDA, 51
Fillers
  bruising from treatments, 216–17
  types
    autologous fat injections, 218–19
    collagen, 213, 215–18, 221
    Restylane, 213, 214–15, 219

  use for
    acne scars, 213, 219
    lip plumping, 220, 221
    static lines, 213
Finacea, for rosacea, 147
Fine lines, treatment of, 220–25
Fitzpatrick skin-typing system, 110
Forehead lines, Botox injections for, 230
Foundation, 176–77
Fragrance
  allergy/reactions to, 59, 151
  removal by All Free Clear laundry detergent, 15
  in shampoo, 172
  in skin-care products, 57, 58
Free radicals, 65
Frizz-Ease Down-Play Volume Reducer, 172
Frontalis muscle, 230
Frown lines
  analyzing in Orientation photos, 23
  Botox injections for, 231
  from strength training, 29

G

Girdle effect, with Botox injections for crow's-feet, 229–30
Glycerin, 58–59, 69
Glycol distearate, 56
Glycolic acid, 130–31, 132
  adverse effects
    broken blood vessels, 155
    irritation and redness from, 151
  benefits of use, 51
  in cleansers, 56
  pH level, 70–71
  in skin-care products, 69–71
  strength of formulation, 51–54, 189
  use for
    crow's-feet, 198
    exfoliation, 69–71, 104, 192, 224
    postinflammatory hyperpigmentation, 136
Glycolic acid peel/wash
  description of, 223
  precautions with, 223–24
  use for
    age spots, 141
    furrowed brow, 197
    melasma, 144
Green tea, 65

H

Hair
  analysis of Orientation photos, 161
  color, 168
  facial, 161–62, 173
  thin, 168–71

S